Current Controversies in the Management of Temporomandibular Disorders

Editors

DANIEL M. LASKIN
SHRAVAN KUMAR RENAPURKAR

ORAL AND MAXILLOFACIAL SURGERY CLINICS OF NORTH AMERICA

www.oralmaxsurgery.theclinics.com

Consulting Editor
RUI P. FERNANDES

August 2018 • Volume 30 • Number 3

ELSEVIER

1600 John F. Kennedy Boulevard • Suite 1800 • Philadelphia, Pennsylvania, 19103-2899

http://www.oralmaxsurgery.theclinics.com

ORAL AND MAXILLOFACIAL SURGERY CLINICS OF NORTH AMERICA Volume 30, Number 3
August 2018 ISSN 1042-3699, ISBN-13: 978-0-323-61404-7

Editor: John Vassallo; j.vassallo@elsevier.com
Developmental Editor: Laura Fisher

Oral and Maxillofacial Surgery Clinics of North America (ISSN 1042-3699) is published quarterly by Elsevier Inc., 360 Park Avenue South, New York, NY 10010-1710. Months of issue are February, May, August, and November. Business and Editorial Offices: 1600 John F. Kennedy Blvd., Suite 1800, Philadelphia, PA 19103-2899. Periodicals postage paid at New York, NY and additional mailing offices. Subscription prices are $393.00 per year for US individuals, $686.00 per year for US institutions, $100.00 per year for US students and residents, $464.00 per year for Canadian individuals, $822.00 per year for Canadian institutions, $520.00 per year for international individuals, $822.00 per year for international institutions and $235.00 per year for Canadian and foreign students/residents. To receive student/resident rate, orders must be accompanied by name or affiliated institution, date of term, and the *signature* of program/residency coordinator on institution letterhead. Orders will be billed at individual rate until proof of status is received. Foreign air speed delivery is included in all *Clinics* subscription prices. All prices are subject to change without notice. **POSTMASTER:** Send address changes to *Oral and Maxillofacial Surgery Clinics of North America,* Elsevier Periodicals **Customer Service, 11830 Westline Industrial Drive, St. Louis, MO 63146. Tel: 1-800-654-2452 (U.S. and Canada); 314-447-8871 (outside U.S. and Canada). Fax: 314-447-8029. E-mail: journals customerservice-usa@elsevier.com (for print support); journalsonlinesupport-usa@elsevier.com (for online support).**

Reprints. For copies of 100 or more, of articles in this publication, please contact the Commercial Reprints Department, Elsevier Inc., 360 Park Avenue South, New York, NY 10010-1710. Tel.: 212-633-3874; Fax: 212-633-3820; Email: reprints@elsevier.com.

Oral and Maxillofacial Surgery Clinics of North America is covered in *MEDLINE/PubMed (Index Medicus), Science Citation Index Expanded (SciSearch®), Journal Citation Reports/Science Edition,* and *Current Contents®/Clinical Medicine.*

Contributors

CONSULTING EDITOR

RUI P. FERNANDES, MD, DMD, FACS, FRCS(Ed)
Clinical Professor and Chief, Division of Head and Neck Surgery, Departments of Oral and Maxillofacial Surgery, Neurosurgery, and Orthopaedic Surgery & Rehabilitation, University of Florida Health Science Center, University of Florida College of Medicine, Jacksonville, FL, USA

EDITORS

DANIEL M. LASKIN, DDS, MS
Professor and Chairman Emeritus, Department of Oral and Maxillofacial Surgery, Virginia Commonwealth University School of Dentistry, Richmond, Virginia, USA

SHRAVAN KUMAR RENAPURKAR, BDS, DMD
Assistant Professor, Department of Oral and Maxillofacial Surgery, Virginia Commonwealth University School of Dentistry, Richmond, Virginia, USA

AUTHORS

LINDA Z. ARVIDSSON, DDS, PhD
Associate Professor, Department of Maxillofacial Radiology, Faculty of Dentistry, Institute of Clinical Dentistry, University of Oslo, Oslo, Norway

GARY F. BOULOUX, MD, DDS, MDSc, FRACDS, FRACDS (OMS), FACS
Professor, Oral and Maxillofacial Surgery, Emory University, Atlanta, Georgia, USA

RADHIKA CHIGURUPATI, DMD, MS
Associate Professor, Department of Oral and Maxillofacial Surgery, Boston University Henry M. Goldman School of Dental Medicine, Boston, Massachusetts, USA

M. FRANKLIN DOLWICK, DMD, PhD
Professor and Chair, Parker E. Mahan Facial Pain Endowed Professor, Department of Oral and Maxillofacial Surgery, University of Florida College of Dentistry, Gainesville, Florida, USA

CHARLES S. GREENE, DDS
Clinical Professor, Department of Orthodontics, UIC College of Dentistry, Chicago, Illinois, USA

GARY M. HEIR, DMD
Professor, Program and Clinical Director, Center for Temporomandibular Disorders and Orofacial Pain, Rutgers School of Dental Medicine, Newark, New Jersey, USA

CAROLINE HOL, DDS
Doctoral Research Fellow, Department of Maxillofacial Radiology, Faculty of Dentistry, Institute of Clinical Dentistry, University of Oslo, Oslo, Norway

DAVID A. KEITH, BDS, DMD
Department of Oral and Maxillofacial Surgery, Massachusetts General Hospital, Boston, Massachusetts, USA

SOMI KIM, DMD, MD
Private Practice, Oral Surgery Partners,
Northborough, Massachusetts, USA

TORE A. LARHEIM, DDS, PhD
Professor, Department of Maxillofacial
Radiology, Faculty of Dentistry, Institute of
Clinical Dentistry, University of Oslo, Oslo,
Norway

DANIEL M. LASKIN, DDS, MS
Professor and Chairman Emeritus, Department
of Oral and Maxillofacial Surgery, Virginia
Commonwealth University School of Dentistry,
Richmond, Virginia, USA

DANIELE MANFREDINI, DDS, MSc, PhD
Department of Medical Biotechnologies,
School of Dental Medicine, University of Siena,
Siena, Italy

PUSHKAR MEHRA, BDS, DMD, FACS
Professor, Chair, Department of Oral and
Maxillofacial Surgery, Boston University Henry
M. Goldman School of Dental Medicine,
Boston, Massachusetts, USA

HAROLD F. MENCHEL, DMD
Adjunct Faculty, Department of
Prosthodontics, Nova Southeastern University
College of Dental Medicine, Davie, Florida,
USA; Private Practice, Coral Springs, Florida,
USA

LOUIS G. MERCURI, DDS, MS
Visiting Professor, Department of Orthopaedic
Surgery, Rush University Medical Center,
Chicago, Illinois, USA; Clinical Consultant,
TMJ Concepts, Ventura, California,
USA

AMBRA MICHELOTTI, BSc, DDS
Department of Neuroscience, Reproductive
Sciences and Oral Sciences, Section of
Orthodontics, University of Naples Federico II,
Naples, Italy

BJØRN B. MORK-KNUTSEN, DDS
Assistant Professor, Department of
Maxillofacial Radiology, Faculty of Dentistry,
Institute of Clinical Dentistry, University of Oslo,
Oslo, Norway

**RICHARD OHRBACH, DDS, PhD,
OdontDr (hon)**
Department of Oral Diagnostic Sciences,
University at Buffalo School of Dental
Medicine, Buffalo, New York, USA

**MARGARETH KRISTENSEN OTTERSEN,
DDS**
Doctoral Research Fellow, Department of
Maxillofacial Radiology, Faculty of Dentistry,
Institute of Clinical Dentistry, University of Oslo,
Oslo, Norway

**SHRAVAN KUMAR RENAPURKAR, BDS,
DMD**
Assistant Professor, Department of Oral and
Maxillofacial Surgery, Virginia Commonwealth
University School of Dentistry, Richmond,
Virginia, USA

BHAVNA SHROFF, DDS, MDentSc, MPA
Professor and Graduate Program Director,
Department of Orthodontics, Virginia
Commonwealth University School of Dentistry,
Richmond, Virginia, USA

CHARLES G. WIDMER, DDS, MS
Associate Professor, Head, Division of Facial
Pain, Department of Orthodontics, University
of Florida College of Dentistry, Gainesville,
Florida, USA

Contents

Introduction   xi

Rui P. Fernandes

Preface: Current Controversies in the Management of Temporomandibular Disorders   xiii

Daniel M. Laskin and Shravan Kumar Renapurkar

The Role of Imaging in the Diagnosis of Temporomandibular Joint Pathology   239

Tore A. Larheim, Caroline Hol, Margareth Kristensen Ottersen, Bjørn B. Mork-Knutsen, and Linda Z. Arvidsson

> Diagnostic imaging is sometimes necessary to supplement the clinical findings in patients with suspected temporomandibular disorders (TMDs). However, the interpretation of pathology in the imaging findings is often complicated by the presence of similar findings in asymptomatic volunteers, as well as by the use of inadequate imaging techniques and poor image quality. This article focuses on these issues and gives guidance on the appropriate use of diagnostic imaging in patients with suspected TMD.

The Use of Synovial Fluid Analysis for Diagnosis of Temporomandibular Joint Disorders   251

Gary F. Bouloux

> There has been considerable progress in the identification of the various synovial fluid cytokines and growth factors associated with various disorders of the temporomandibular joint. However, the presence of the same inflammatory mediators and proteins in these conditions, despite differing causes, makes it very difficult to identify the specific disease using synovial fluid analysis alone.

Occlusal Equilibration for the Management of Temporomandibular Disorders   257

Daniele Manfredini

> The concept of equilibrating the occlusion to treat and/or to prevent temporomandibular disorders found its background in the old precepts of gnathology, but an assessment of the available literature as well as an appraisal of its biological rationale suggests that it is not recommended for routine use.

The Use of Oral Appliances in the Management of Temporomandibular Disorders   265

Charles S. Greene and Harold F. Menchel

> Oral appliances (OAs) are widely used for treating various types of temporomandibular disorders (TMDs); however, many controversies persist about how they should be designed, how they should be used, and even what their ultimate purpose might be. This article discusses 6 of the current controversies, with a focus on the evidence available to support reasonable practice guidelines for the clinical use of OAs in treating certain TMDs.

The Efficacy of Pharmacologic Treatment of Temporomandibular Disorders   279

Gary M. Heir

> This article is not a pharmacopeia offering directions for choosing the proper pain medication for treating temporomandibular disorders. Rather, the appropriate

decision depends on proper diagnosis, an understanding of the pain mechanisms involved, and the different targets for analgesic action. This article discusses these issues and evaluates the various drugs involved. It also describes potential reasons for therapeutic failure.

The Use of Botulinum Toxin for the Treatment of Myofascial Pain in the Masticatory Muscles   287

Daniel M. Laskin

Although the use of botulinum toxin has been recommended for the management of myofascial pain and dysfunction, the precise mechanism of its action remains undetermined and studies on its effectiveness are equivocal. Moreover, even if such treatment may temporarily relieve the symptoms, it does not address the cause of the problem. Also, its use is not free of potential complications. On this basis, botulinum toxin does not seem to be a logical treatment of myofascial pain and dysfunction.

Surgical Versus Nonsurgical Management of Degenerative Joint Disease   291

Shravan Kumar Renapurkar

As knowledge of the complexity of myofascial pain and its interaction with temporomandibular joint disorders has increased, the use of surgical procedures to treat degenerative joint disease has decreased. The focus has moved from a "surgery-first" approach toward a more cautious one that involves nonsurgical treatment as the primary modality, then minimally invasive treatments, followed by open surgical modalities, when indicated. This article examines the current literature regarding the effectiveness of nonsurgical and surgical treatments for the management of degenerative joint disease.

Malocclusion as a Cause for Temporomandibular Disorders and Orthodontics as a Treatment   299

Bhavna Shroff

This article explores the long-standing controversy between orthodontics and temporomandibular disorders (TMDs). It reviews the history of this controversy and presents a discussion of the current literature concerning the potential role of malocclusion in the onset of TMDs. It also explores the potential role of orthodontic treatment as a possible cure for TMDs and concludes, based on the most current evidence-based literature, that there is no relationship.

Orthognathic Surgery as a Treatment for Temporomandibular Disorders   303

M. Franklin Dolwick and Charles G. Widmer

Well-controlled clinical trials supporting orthognathic surgery as the primary management for temporomandibular disorders (TMDs) are lacking. Most published studies lack an adequate experimental design to minimize biases. Studies that did minimize some biases do support an overall reduction in the frequency of TMD signs and symptoms in some class III and class II patients who had orthognathic surgery. However, class II correction with counterclockwise rotation of the mandible increased TMD. Individual variability precludes the ability to predict TMD outcome after surgery. Irreversible therapies such as orthognathic surgery should not be primary treatments in the management or prevention of TMDs.

Arthroscopy Versus Arthrocentesis for Treating Internal Derangements of the Temporomandibular Joint   325

Daniel M. Laskin

The introduction of arthroscopy of the temporomandibular joint represented a major change in the management of internal derangements and led to the realization that reestablishing joint mobility by arthroscopic lysis and lavage was as effective as surgically restoring disc position. It was subsequently shown that such treatment could be done without joint visualization, which raised the question of whether the inability to visualize the joint and perform other surgical manipulations limited its usefulness. A comparison of the literature shows that, although their effectiveness is essentially the same, arthrocentesis is simpler, has less morbidity, and has fewer complications than arthroscopic surgery.

Discectomy Versus Disc Preservation for Internal Derangement of the Temporomandibular Joint   329

Shravan Kumar Renapurkar

Anterior disc displacement with or without reduction is a common finding in symptomatic and asymptomatic individuals. When symptomatic and associated with dysfunction it requires an intervention. Once nonsurgical management fails and the patient does not respond to minimally invasive procedures, open surgical treatment is indicated. However, controversy exists about whether disc-preservation procedures, such as repositioning/repairing or disc removal, are the preferred treatment. This article evaluates the current evidence supporting both treatment options and highlights the indications, contraindications, and consequences of each.

Costochondral Graft Versus Total Alloplastic Joint for Temporomandibular Joint Reconstruction   335

Louis G. Mercuri

There are 2 options for the replacement of the temporomandibular joint for end-stage pathology: autogenous bone grafting or alloplastic joint replacement. This article presents evidence-based advantages and disadvantages for each of these management options to assist both surgeons and their patients in making that choice.

Injectable Agents Versus Surgery for Recurrent Temporomandibular Joint Dislocation   343

Shravan Kumar Renapurkar and Daniel M. Laskin

Recurrent temporomandibular joint dislocation (TMJD) is a distressing entity to the patient and a therapeutic challenge to the treating provider. Absence of high-level evidence in the literature among currently available treatment options creates a lack of consistency in management. This article reviews the current literature on common injectable agents used and the open surgical techniques. Based on the findings, an injectable agent is the initial treatment of choice for recurrent TMJD, with capsulorraphy and eminectomy being used in nonresponding patients.

Combined or Staged Temporomandibular Joint and Orthognathic Surgery for Patients with Internal Derangement and Dentofacial Deformities   351

Somi Kim and David A. Keith

Patients with internal derangement of the temporomandibular joint and dentofacial deformities need appropriate evaluation for both conditions. Correct diagnosis of internal derangement is vital in determining the correct orthognathic surgery plan, and it is particularly important to differentiate between myofascial dysfunction and intraarticular joint problems. Depending on the stage of internal derangement, patients may need treatment for temporomandibular dysfunction symptomatically, staged, or concurrently with orthognathic surgery.

Surgical Management of Idiopathic Condylar Resorption: Orthognathic Surgery Versus Temporomandibular Total Joint Replacement

355

Radhika Chigurupati and Pushkar Mehra

Young women with retruded and hyperdivergent mandibles, class II open-bite malocclusions, and steep occlusal planes with or without temporomandibular joint symptoms are at higher risk for idiopathic condylar resorption (ICR). Such patients undergoing orthodontic and/or surgical treatment should be informed of possible relapse due to ICR. Orthognathic surgery with total joint replacement or orthognathic surgery alone may both be acceptable options for the management of the facial deformity and the malocclusion that ensues from ICR. Proper patient selection is key to achieving a successful outcome. Current trends and the evidence in the literature suggest that orthognathic surgery with alloplastic joint replacement may be the preferred approach.

The Role of Stress in the Etiology of Oral Parafunction and Myofascial Pain

369

Richard Ohrbach and Ambra Michelotti

Oral parafunction during waking comprises possible behaviors that can be measured with a comprehensive checklist or behavioral monitoring. Multiple studies lead to largely consistent findings: stressful states can trigger parafunctional episodes that contribute to myofascial pain. However, this simple causal pathway coexists with at least 3 other pathways: anxiety and stress are potent direct contributors to pain, pain results in maladaptive behaviors such as parafunction, and parafunction may be a coping response to potential threat coupled with hypervigilance and somatosensory amplification. Awake parafunction remains an important risk factor for myofascial pain onset, and overuse models alone of causation are insufficient.

ORAL AND MAXILLOFACIAL SURGERY CLINICS OF NORTH AMERICA

FORTHCOMING ISSUES

November 2018
The Head and Neck Cancer Patient: Perioperative Care and Assessment
Zvonimir L. Milas and Thomas D. Shellenberger, *Editors*

February 2019
The Head and Neck Cancer Patient: Treatment
Zvonimir L. Milas and Thomas D. Shellenberger, *Editors*

May 2019
Dental Implants, Part I: Reconstruction
Ole Jensen, *Editor*

RECENT ISSUES

May 2018
Anesthesia
David W. Todd and Robert C. Bosack, *Editors*

February 2018
Pediatric Temporomandibular Joint Disorders
Shelly Abramowicz, *Editor*

November 2017
Controversies in Oral and Maxillofacial Surgery
Luis G. Vega and Daniel J. Meara, *Editors*

SERIES OF RELATED INTEREST

Atlas of the Oral and Maxillofacial Surgery Clinics
www.oralmaxsurgeryatlas.theclinics.com

Dental Clinics
www.dental.theclinics.com

THE CLINICS ARE NOW AVAILABLE ONLINE!
Access your subscription at:
www.theclinics.com

Introduction

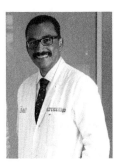

Rui P. Fernandes, MD, DMD, FACS, FRCS(Ed)
Consulting Editor

In modern academic medicine, seldom do we see longevity. Richard Haug was an exception. He served as the Consulting Editor of *Oral and Maxillofacial Surgery Clinics of North America* for nearly 15 years, truly a phenomenal accomplishment. During this time, he oversaw numerous *Oral and Maxillofacial Surgery Clinics of North America* issues and worked with countless editors and contributing authors. His dedication to this publication was evident to all of us who had the opportunity to work with him, as he set the standard for what the *Oral and Maxillofacial Surgery Clinics of North America* is today.

I am humbled today to introduce myself as the new Consulting Editor of the *Oral and Maxillofacial Surgery Clinics of North America*, a recommendation made to the publisher by Rich prior to his untimely death this past year. I am excited and eager to take on this challenge. I look forward to working with future guest editors and contributing authors and will do my utmost to build upon the strong foundation that Dr Haug has provided.

Rui P. Fernandes, MD, DMD, FACS, FRCS(Ed)
Division of Head and Neck Surgery
Departments of OMFS, Neurosurgery
Orthopedic Surgery
University of Florida College of Medicine
Jacksonville
653-1 West 8th Street
Jacksonville, FL 32209, USA

E-mail address:
rui.fernandes@jax.ufl.edu

Oral Maxillofacial Surg Clin N Am 30 (2018) xi
https://doi.org/10.1016/j.coms.2018.06.002
1042-3699/18/© 2018 Published by Elsevier Inc.

Preface

Current Controversies in the Management of Temporomandibular Disorders

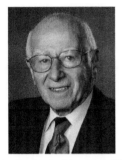
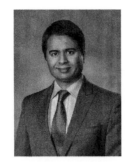

Daniel M. Laskin, DDS, MS   Shravan Kumar Renapurkar, BDS, DMD
Editors

Despite many years of both basic and clinical research in the field, clinicians continue to have difficulty adequately managing many of the various temporomandibular disorders. This is due in part to the conflicting information and differing opinions found in the literature. This includes etiologic and diagnostic issues as well as those related to therapeutic decisions. As a result, patients do not always receive the most appropriate treatment. It is the intent of this issue to resolve some of these most controversial issues. To accomplish this, experts in the various areas were asked to address the selected subjects based solely on their evaluation of the best evidence available in the literature. However, in considering the conclusions reached by the authors, the reader should consider that "best evidence" in some of the areas is not always best, and that this will be reflected in the conclusions provided. The answers provided may still offer some guidance to the reader, but such areas will need further investigation before more definitive answers can be derived.

We would like to thank the various contributors for their time and effort in helping make this issue possible. It is our hope that their efforts will be a step forward toward further improving patient care in this complex field.

Daniel M. Laskin, DDS, MS
Department of Oral and Maxillofacial Surgery
Virginia Commonwealth University
School of Dentistry
521 North 11th Street
Richmond, VA 23298-0566, USA

Shravan Kumar Renapurkar, BDS, DMD
Department of Oral and Maxillofacial Surgery
Virginia Commonwealth University
School of Dentistry
521 North 11th Street
Richmond, VA 23298-0566, USA

E-mail addresses:
dmlaskin@vcu.edu (D.M. Laskin)
srenapurkar@vcu.edu (S.K. Renapurkar)

Oral Maxillofacial Surg Clin N Am 30 (2018) xiii
https://doi.org/10.1016/j.coms.2018.05.005
1042-3699/18/© 2018 Published by Elsevier Inc.

The Role of Imaging in the Diagnosis of Temporomandibular Joint Pathology

Tore A. Larheim, DDS, PhD*, Caroline Hol, DDS,
Margareth Kristensen Ottersen, DDS,
Bjørn B. Mork-Knutsen, DDS, Linda Z. Arvidsson, DDS, PhD

KEYWORDS

- Diagnostic imaging • Temporomandibular joint disorders • Temporomandibular joint disc
- Osteoarthritis • Cone-beam computed tomography (CBCT) • Computed tomography • MRI

KEY POINTS

- The reliability of temporomandibular joint imaging increases with optimized image quality, calibrated/experienced observers, and a focus on frank pathologic findings not reported in asymptomatic volunteers.
- The presence of intraarticular disc displacement may not always represent pathology.
- Joint effusion should be considered pathologic only if there is more fluid than reported in asymptomatic volunteers. Coexistence with bone marrow edema indicates a more pronounced inflammatory reaction.
- The diagnosis of osteoarthritis should be based on evident abnormalities, in particular bone destruction, and not on subtle changes that may represent a normal anatomic variation or remodeling.
- Panoramic radiographs are only reliable for imaging gross bony changes in the condyle.

INTRODUCTION

Clinical examination sometimes provides limited information with respect to the joint status in patients with temporomandibular disorder (TMD).[1] Therefore, diagnostic imaging is often necessary to reliably assess the temporomandibular joints (TMJs). However, there is a controversy as to what should be classified as joint pathology. It is also a fact that observer performance may be highly variable and that image quality may vary considerably in routine clinical practice. To assess TMJ pathology it is also mandatory to know the range of normalcy, that is, imaging signs observed in healthy individuals. This review focuses on the accuracy of the diagnostic interpretation of disc displacement, joint effusion, and osteoarthritis in the TMJ and common errors that are made in image interpretation.

DISC DISPLACEMENT
Is Disc Displacement a Normal Condition?

Before the era of diagnostic imaging, displacement of the articular disc relative to the mandibular condyle was diagnosed based on symptoms such

Disclosure Statement: The authors have nothing to disclose.
Department of Maxillofacial Radiology, Faculty of Dentistry, Institute of Clinical Dentistry, University of Oslo, PO Box 1109, Blindern, Oslo 0317, Norway
* Corresponding author.
E-mail address: t.a.larheim@odont.uio.no

Oral Maxillofacial Surg Clin N Am 30 (2018) 239–249
https://doi.org/10.1016/j.coms.2018.04.001

as clicking sounds and impaired mouth opening.[2] When soft-tissue imaging of the TMJ became possible, displacement of the disc was frequently confirmed in such patients[3] and was considered to be the main cause of the pain.[4] However, when MRI was performed on persons without TMD, some disc displacement was found in as many as one-third of them.[5–7] Thus, there is still a controversy over when disc displacement is a pathologic condition and when it is a normal variant.[5,8]

Are There Differences Between Symptomatic Patients and Asymptomatic Volunteers Regarding Disc Displacement?

In studies of asymptomatic volunteers the anteriorly displaced disc has been found to reduce on open-mouth images in almost all joints examined.[5–7,9–11] Moreover, Larheim and colleagues[7] reported that 90% of the displaced discs in volunteers were only partially displaced, supporting a study of Rammelsberg and colleagues.[11] The same observation was made in a study of schoolchildren without symptoms.[12] All these studies indicate that partial anterior disc displacement most frequently occurs in the lateral portion of the disc. On the other hand, complete disc displacement, that is, a disc that is anteriorly displaced in all sections through the joint, is almost only observed in symptomatic patients.[7] Such findings indicate the need to correlate the clinical symptoms with the imaging findings in determining whether a partially displaced disc is the cause of a patient's problems. **Fig. 1** shows a partially displaced disc in an asymptomatic volunteer and a completely displaced disc in a symptomatic patient.

Is Imaging Diagnosis of Disc Displacement Reliable?

In a systematic review by Limchaichana and colleagues,[13] the sensitivity and specificity, as well as observer performance of diagnosing disc position by imaging, varied considerably and the investigators concluded that the evidence for diagnostic efficacy was insufficient. In a study comparing sagittal MRI sections and cryosections of autopsy TMJ specimens, the sensitivity and

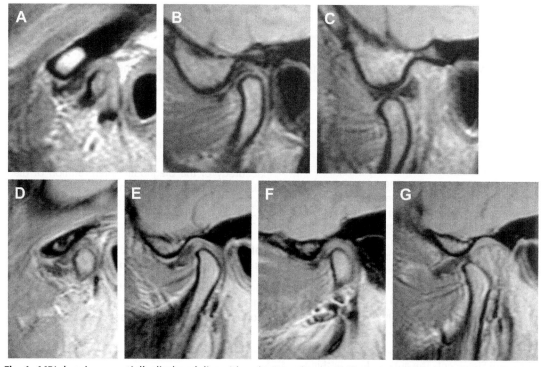

Fig. 1. MRI showing a partially displaced disc with reduction: the disc is displaced anteriorly in the lateral part of the joint (*A*) but normally located in the centromedial part in the closed-mouth position (*B*), and normally located in the open-mouth position (*C*). MRI showing a completely displaced disc without reduction: the disc is anteriorly displaced in all sections throughout the joint in the closed mouth (*D–F*) and open mouth positions (*G*). (*Adapted from* Larheim TA, Westesson P, Sano T. Temporomandibular joint disk displacement: comparison in asymptomatic volunteers and patients. Radiology 2001;218(2):430–1; with permission.)

specificity in identifying an anterior disc position were 0.86 and 0.63, respectively.[14] Studies comparing the combination of sagittal and coronal MR sections were only better for specificity, with sensitivities and specificities of 0.87 and 0.80[15] and 0.75 and 0.92, respectively.[16] However, in a more recent study, Tasaki and Westesson[17] obtained a diagnostic accuracy of 95% in the assessment of disc position. The higher reliability than in previous studies was explained by improved quality of the MR images,[18] as well as a greater observer experience in interpreting the images.

The quality of the MR images has been shown to have an impact on the observer performance. In one study, the level of interobserver agreement was low with mean kappa values ranging from 0.27 to 0.38 in 5 different diagnostic TMJ criteria assessed before the selection of the high-quality image sets.[19] The strength of agreement was only fair (kappa 0.21–0.40) according to Altman.[20] When the diagnosis was based on the high-quality images, the mean kappa values increased to 0.43 to 0.55, which is moderate strength of agreement. This is an important issue that has not received much attention. In routine clinical practice the quality of TMJ MRIs is highly variable.

There are also huge observer differences in the diagnostic assessment of various grades of the disc position. Using a combination of oblique sagittal and coronal images, interobserver agreement was lowest (kappa 0.19) for the diagnosis of slight anterior disc displacement. In contrast, the highest kappa value was 0.91, obtained for disc displacement without reduction.[21] Thus, the strength of agreement ranged from poor (kappa ≤ 0.20) to very good (kappa 0.81–1.00).[20] A very good interobserver agreement (kappa 0.94) for diagnosing disc displacement without reduction was also found by Ahmad and colleagues.[22] The high interobserver agreement makes the imaging diagnosis of disc displacement without reduction more reliable than for other types of disc displacement.

It is not surprising that the interobserver agreement in the assessment of slight disc displacement in closed-mouth images is low. High-signal-intensity areas on MRI occasionally occur in the posterior band in a normal joint,[23,24] making it difficult to precisely determine the border between the low-signal posterior band and the high-signal posterior attachment. Moreover, variations of the posterior band position in joints with normal disc position have been found in different individuals.[10] Further, the definition of a normal disc position is controversial because different methods to quantify the disc position have been applied.[11]

Although attempts have been made to define the normal range,[24] there is no overall consensus as to how much displacement is considered abnormal.[25] Thus, there are good reasons to conclude that disc positions slightly different from the 12-o'clock position in closed-mouth images should be considered within normalcy.

Is Disc Displacement Related to Osteoarthritis?

In numerous studies, disc displacement and osteoarthritis are coexisting, and this association has been demonstrated both in clinical studies and in autopsy materials.[26] However, it is controversial whether disc displacement leads to osteoarthritis or vice versa. In joints with disc displacement without reduction and normal cortical bone at baseline, osteoarthritis has been demonstrated to develop over time.[26] In a recent longitudinal study of 401 persons, the authors concluded that osteoarthritis could be a result of, or a precursor for, disc displacement.[27] This has also been suggested by other investigators.[28] In joints with evident bone-destructive changes and a normally located disc, a traumatic cause or rheumatic disease should be suspected. In inflammatory arthritis the disc is most frequently located in a normal position.[29]

Is Disc Displacement Always Symptomatic?

A recent, comprehensive review concluded that many investigators have reported anterior disc displacement as an important source of joint pain, particularly in joints without disc reduction.[30] This study substantiated a previous systematic literature review, in which the calculated odds ratio for the relationship between pain and disc displacement without reduction was high.[31] On the other hand, it was also stated that some investigators have demonstrated that anterior disc displacement without reduction does not necessarily correlate with joint pain. The relationship between lateral or medial disc displacement and joint pain has also yielded controversial results.[30]

As evidenced from the literature, disc displacement without reduction seems to be more related to joint pain than other types of disc displacement. However, it is not the displaced disc per se that seems to be responsible for the symptoms but rather the functional disturbance.

JOINT EFFUSION

Joint fluid or effusion in the TMJ appears as an area of high T2 signal intensity in the joint compartments.[32] The terms fluid and effusion are used interchangeably, although in some studies effusion is used for an abnormal amount of fluid.

How Is Joint Effusion Defined and How Frequently Is It Seen?

MRI evidence of joint effusion was recognized in one of the earliest TMJ studies using surface coil technology.[33] Later studies have shown that effusion is found particularly in joints with a displaced disc.[26] However, the frequency of joint effusion reported in patients with TMD has varied substantially. Manfredini and colleagues[34] reported a frequency of 20% to 26%, whereas Westesson and Brooks[32] and Rudisch and colleagues[35] reported frequencies of 40% to 50% and 60%, respectively. A frequency of up to 88% also has been published[36] but without comparison with observations in healthy individuals. In most of these studies the joints showed disc displacement.

Westesson and Brooks[32] regarded lack of a high T2 signal or a line of high signal along the articular surface to be normal and joint effusion to be present when more than a line was observed. This definition was adopted by others[37] but was modified by Emshoff and colleagues[38] who proposed that more than a line of high signal had to be evident on at least 2 consecutive T2 sections. Manfredini and colleagues[34] considered effusion in the joint compartment to be present when the high T2 signal exceeded 2 mm. According to Ahmad and colleagues,[22] slight effusion meant a bright signal in either joint space that conformed to the contours of the disc, fossa/articular eminence, and/or condyle, and frank effusion extended beyond the osseous contours of the fossa/articular eminence and/or condyle with a convex configuration in the anterior or posterior recess.

The large range of frequency can at least partly be explained by the different definitions of TMJ effusion being used.

Are There Differences Between Patients and Asymptomatic Volunteers Regarding Joint Effusion and What Is an Abnormal Amount of Fluid?

A comprehensive study of asymptomatic volunteers was performed by Larheim and colleagues[39] who examined a group of 62 asymptomatic individuals. Lines or dots of high T2 signal along the articular surface, defined as minimal fluid, were observed in 34%. A larger amount, categorized as moderate fluid, was observed in 19%. Thus, 53% of the asymptomatic volunteers had MR evidence of joint fluid. The fluid was usually observed

laterally in the anterior recess of the upper joint compartment and was consistently related to an anterior disc displacement. By comparison, 69% of 58 patients with TMD in the same study showed no or minimal fluid, whereas the remaining 31% had a larger amount. However, only about 10% in the entire series of patients had an amount of fluid that was greater than that seen in any of the asymptomatic volunteers. **Fig. 2** shows fluid in an asymptomatic volunteer and effusion in a symptomatic patient.

The challenge of defining an abnormal amount of fluid is the same for any joint, and knowledge about fluid in healthy individuals is mandatory in order to define pathology. In a study of the knee, the investigators concluded that joint effusion should be recorded only when the amount of fluid exceeded the maximum amount observed in the asymptomatic volunteers.[40] Using this definition, based on the findings of TMJ fluid observed in 62 asymptomatic volunteers,[39] TMJ effusion was found in 70 patients (13%) in a series of 523 consecutively examined patients with TMD.[41]

It is difficult to arrive at a conclusion of what should be considered an abnormal amount of TMJ fluid but, as suggested in the literature, this should be judged based on reported observations in asymptomatic volunteers.

How Is Joint Fluid Graded and Is Such Grading Reliable?

Different systems for grading TMJ fluid have been proposed. The one proposed by Larheim and colleagues[41] consisted of no, minimal, moderate, and marked fluid, and recently has been used by several others.[42,43] In this system, minimal fluid is not regarded as an abnormality. However, other investigators have classified minimal or mild joint fluid as an abnormal finding,[44] or they have used the grading system of Ahmad and colleagues,[22] which classifies slight or minimal fluid as an abnormal amount.[45]

Little attention has been given to the observer performance in the diagnostic assessment of joint effusion. In the study by Takano and colleagues,[46] observer agreement among 7 noncalibrated observers showed an overall kappa of only 0.36, that is, the strength of agreement was fair, and the values were even lower for the different categories. The kappa value increased to 0.52, a moderate strength of agreement, when the categories were dichotomized to presence or absence of joint fluid.[46] From these studies it can be concluded that there is considerable variation among observers regarding the grading of effusion and care needs to be taken in the clinical significance

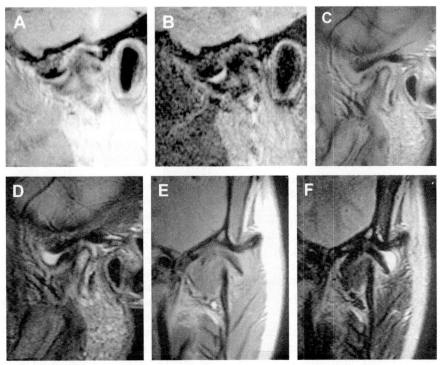

Fig. 2. MRI showing joint fluid in the anterior recess of upper joint compartment (*A, B*). These images demonstrate the maximum amount of fluid observed in a series of asymptomatic volunteers. MRI showing an abnormal amount of fluid, that is, joint effusion in the anterolateral recess of upper joint compartment (*C–F*). (*Adapted from* Larheim TA, Katzberg RW, Westesson PL, et al. MR evidence of temporomandibular joint fluid and condyle marrow alterations: occurrence in asymptomatic volunteers and symptomatic patients. Int J Oral Maxillofac Surg 2001;30(2):115; with permission; and Larheim TA. Role of magnetic resonance imaging in the clinical diagnosis of the temporomandibular joint. Cells Tissues Organs 2005;180(1):14; with permission.)

placed on such findings, particularly when the amount of fluid is minimal.

Are Disc Displacement and Joint Effusion Related?

Joint effusion is frequently found in joints of patients with TMD with disc displacement.[26] Manfredini and colleagues[34] found a significant relationship between effusion and disc displacement without reduction, but not between effusion and disc displacement with reduction. In another study, two-thirds of 76 joints with unquestionable effusion had disc displacement without reduction.[41] Ahmad and colleagues[22] stated that "it is now understood that effusion occurs with disc displacement," by referring to Westesson and Brooks[32] and Larheim and colleagues.[41]

Is Joint Effusion Related to Osteoarthritis?

Joint effusion is found both in joints with normal bony structure and in joints with osteoarthritis. In the analyses of 76 joints with unquestionable effusion, Larheim and colleagues[41] found that about 60% had normal cortical bone and 40% had

osteoarthritis. This observation supported that of Westesson and Brooks[32] who also found that the frequency of joint effusion was lower in joints with osteoarthritis than in those with disc displacement and normal bone. Because joint effusion occurs both in joints with and without osteoarthritis one needs to be cautious in using it as a diagnostic criterion for this condition.

Is Joint Effusion Related to Abnormal Bone Marrow?

Larheim and colleagues[47] found that 39% (7 of 18 cases) with histologically documented marrow edema and/or osteonecrosis in the mandibular condyle showed signs of joint effusion on MRI. This is in accordance with MRI observations in various stages of osteonecrosis of the hip.[48] The association between TMJ effusion and abnormal bone marrow has also been observed in clinical MRI studies.[36,49,50] In a selective group of 76 joints with unquestionable effusion, the majority had disc displacement without reduction and one-fourth had abnormal bone marrow.[41] The presence of joint effusion in joints with bone marrow edema indicates a more pronounced inflammatory reaction than if effusion occurs without abnormal marrow.

Is Joint Effusion Related to Joint Pain?

Some investigators have reported a relationship between joint effusion and joint pain (spontaneous and/or provoked), whereas others have not reported such a relationship.[31] These conflicting results have been confirmed in a recent review.[30] Moreover, in a report by Khawaja and colleagues,[45] no association was found between joint effusion and pain, whereas Takahara and colleagues[42] reported an association between joint pain and anterior disc displacement without reduction, severe bony changes, joint effusion, and bone marrow edema. Although more investigators have reported a positive relationship between joint effusion and joint pain than those who have not, the relationship between joint effusion and joint pain still remains unclear.

Variations in Joint Fluid over Time

Whereas disc displacement and osteoarthritis remained stable in more than 70% of patients with TMD during an 8-year follow-up study,[27] reports have suggested that other variables such as joint effusion may fluctuate over time. In a case report on inflammatory TMJ arthritis followed for about 16 months, the amount of joint effusion (and marrow edema) changed, reflecting exacerbation and subsidence of the inflammation.[51] The cyclic changes corresponded well with the pain experience. Another longitudinal study of patients with TMD with disc displacement also showed variations in TMJ fluid and pain during the observation period.[52] In a recent 3-year follow-up study of untreated disc displacement without reduction, a significant decrease in the amount of joint effusion was observed.[53] Finally, also in a long-term follow-up, Bristela and colleagues[54] showed that the number of joints with effusion gradually reduced, although not significantly. Two-thirds of the patients who had pain at baseline became pain free. These studies seem to show that joint effusion fluctuates when followed longitudinally.

In summary, joint effusion can be considered pathologic if the amount of fluid is greater than that reported in asymptomatic volunteers. However, because the amount of fluid in the joint can fluctuate over time, it is not a good indicator of joint pathology.

OSTEOARTHRITIS

This is the most frequent intraarticular osseous abnormality found in patients with TMD referred for diagnostic imaging. Because clinical examination for diagnosing osteoarthritis has low sensitivity (0.55) and specificity (0.61) with computed tomography (CT) as a reference method,[1] imaging is needed for reliable diagnoses.

Which Is the Best Imaging Method for Bony Changes?

For decades MRI has been recommended and used for examination of the TMJs in patients with TMD.[26] It has been the primary imaging method because it is the only method that can visualize both soft tissue and bone. However, for bone examination, CT is in general accepted as superior to MRI at least regarding bone surface abnormalities. In the comprehensive study of diagnostic imaging criteria, Ahmad and colleagues[22] compared panoramic and MRI examinations with CT for assessing their validity for detecting osteoarthritis. The interobserver reliability (with 3 observers) for diagnosing osteoarthritis was poor when based on the panoramic images (kappa 0.16), better when based on MRI (kappa 0.47), and clearly better when based on CT (kappa 0.71). The results indicated that about 40% of CT-diagnosed osteoarthritis was not detected with MRI.

It has been convincingly shown that the accuracy of cone beam computed tomography (CBCT) for TMJ diagnostics is comparable with regular CT and with a lower radiation dose.[55] CBCT has an acceptable accuracy for diagnosing osseous abnormalities with fairly high sensitivity (in the range 0.7–0.9), although smaller cortical defects might be missed. In most studies, high specificity was also reported.[55] However, it must be emphasized that there are differences between CBCT machines regarding image quality.

CT is an excellent imaging modality to visualize the cortical bone abnormalities that characterize TMJ osteoarthritis,[56,57] and CT definitions for surface erosion, subcortical cysts, osteophytes, and sclerosis have been published.[22] These diagnostic criteria can surely be applied to CBCT images as well.[55]

In general, bone-productive changes usually dominate in osteoarthritis.[58] However, although erosions are not typical, they may be a dominant feature of the disease both in the TMJ and in other joints. However, it is unclear how pronounced the changes must be to be classified as disease.[22] This concerns both bone-productive and bone-destructive changes. It can be a challenge to differentiate between morphologic variations of normalcy and small pathologic changes, such as between subtle "beaking" of the anterior aspect of the condyle and a small osteophyte.[55]

Moreover, small osteophytelike formations have been reported in asymptomatic individuals,[59,60] and an osteophytelike appearance on CBCT images can even be created by motion artifacts.[55] **Fig. 3** indicates the challenge of differentiating between normalcy and pathology.

In previous MRI studies of asymptomatic volunteers, cortical irregularities in the TMJ were found in less than 3%.[10,59,60] However, in CBCT studies more variable and much higher frequencies have been reported, up to nearly 80%.[61–63] Using CBCT, which is superior to MRI for diagnosing bony details, subtler changes can be recognized. Recently, TMJ osteoarthritis was found in 67% in a cohort of patients with hand osteoarthritis.[61] It must be considered controversial that this frequency is lower than that reported in one of the studies of asymptomatic individuals. The extreme differences in frequency in the CBCT studies of asymptomatic individuals are difficult to explain. However, based on some of the illustrations in these articles, there should be more focus on image quality and understanding of the diagnostic criteria.

With the increasing use of CBCT another challenge may arise. More TMJs will most likely be scanned, both intentionally and unintentionally, using equipment with a large field of view. The probability of "detecting" morphologic deviations will thus increase. It is very important not to focus on such deviations in individuals without any subjective complaints.

The bone marrow cannot be evaluated by imaging methods other than MRI. The normal marrow signal is homogeneous[47]; signal heterogeneity is not reported in asymptomatic volunteers.[39] Bone marrow edema is characterized by an increased signal on T2 images and reduced signal on T1 or proton density images.[47] When compared with histology, MRI is fairly insensitive in the detection of marrow edema in the mandibular condyle.[47] This is similar to an experimental study of marrow edema in the femoral head.[62] Further, a poor agreement has been reported when noncalibrated observers are diagnosing bone marrow edema.[46] Obviously, it is difficult to decide what an increased signal and a decreased signal are in the condyle marrow.

Osteonecrosis should be suspected when bone marrow edema occurs simultaneously with a low signal on all sequences consistent with marrow sclerosis or fibrosis.[47] The diagnosis of osteonecrosis in the TMJ was controversial until it was histologically documented, apparently as a separate entity but also in advanced osteoarthritis. It is now included in the expanded diagnostic criteria/TMD.[63] As marrow edema, osteonecrosis can probably be a precursor for osteoarthritis.[47] However, distinguishing osteonecrosis from osteoarthritis on imaging can be impossible.

It is evident from the literature that CBCT (or CT) is the most reliable imaging method for the diagnostic assessment of osteoarthritis, although the bone marrow cannot be evaluated as it can be with MRI. The focus should not be on subtle changes that may be seen frequently in asymptomatic volunteers, but on evident changes, in particular bone destruction.

Is Panoramic Imaging of Value for Examination of the Temporomandibular Joints for Bony Changes?

In a study comparing panoramic radiography and MRI with CT, about 75% of CT-assessed osteoarthritis was not detected with panoramic radiography.[22] The interobserver reliability was also poor, supporting previous studies.[64–66] A position paper by the American Academy of Oral and Maxillofacial Radiology indicates that panoramic radiography is useful to detect gross TMJ pathology.[67] **Fig. 4** shows no clear TMJ pathology on the panoramic image, but osteoarthritis is visible on the CBCT sections. However, only the mandibular condyle, and not the glenoid fossa, can be evaluated on panoramic images. Further, the anatomy of the condyle, in particular the angulation of the long axis, which may vary considerably both intraindividually and interindividually, can have a great impact on the panoramic appearance. A gracile but normal condyle as seen on CBCT, with a large angulation of the long axis, may have an appearance that easily can be misinterpreted as a deformation on a panoramic image.

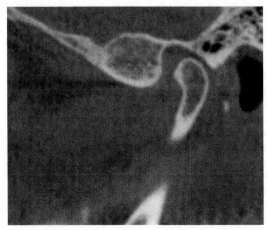

Fig. 3. CBCT showing the difficulty in distinguishing normal anatomy from an osteophyte of the condyle.

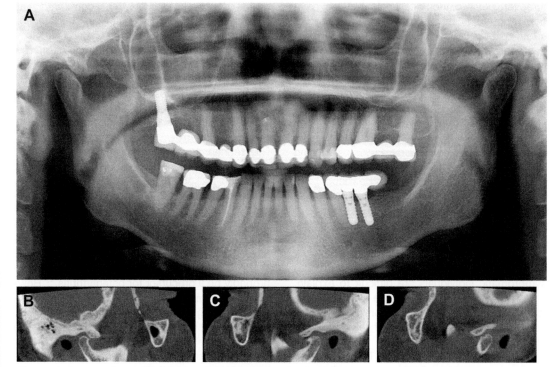

Fig. 4. Panoramic radiograph indicates a normal right condyle and some sclerosis in the left condyle (*A*). CBCT of the same patient shows a normal right condyle (*B*) but an evident osteophyte/sclerosis and cortical defect in the left condyle (*C, D*).

It can be concluded that panoramic imaging may detect large abnormalities of the mandibular condyle but minor abnormalities can easily be missed. The shape of the condyle should be considered with caution with regard to normalcy versus pathology.

SUMMARY

Misdiagnosis is a major problem in the treatment of patients with TMD, in particular in the differentiation between extraarticular and intraarticular causes of pain and dysfunction.[68] The importance of a thorough clinical examination cannot be stressed enough. When an intraarticular condition is suspected as the main cause of pain and dysfunction, it is crucial that imaging demonstrates TMJ pathology before any invasive joint treatment is initiated. From this review it should be clear that the changes in the TMJ must be different or more pronounced than those observed in asymptomatic volunteers. Subtle changes should receive little attention because they may represent anatomic variations. Classifying such changes as pathology can lead to overdiagnosis. Moreover, it is evident from the literature that observer agreement when diagnosing subtle changes is often very low. This is in contrast to more evident TMJ pathology, such as disc displacement without reduction, in which there is very high observer agreement. When a functional joint disturbance is accompanied by inflammatory reactions such as joint effusion and bone marrow edema, the TMJ pathology is even more obvious. However, as with disc position diagnostics, there should be no focus on subtle findings.

To perform both soft tissue and bone diagnostics simultaneously, MRI is the only valid imaging method. According to the diagnostic criteria/ TMD, the clinical diagnosis of disc displacement without reduction is very reliable when mouth opening is impaired. Therefore, in such cases, there may be no need for MRI but rather CBCT or CT assessment of the bony structures.

It is evident from the literature that imaging signs can be dynamic. Although stability regarding both disc displacement and osteoarthritis seems to be most common, both progression and reversal do occur. Also subjective symptoms such as pain may fluctuate over time. If the clinician is in doubt with regard to the management of a patient, follow-up imaging could be a possibility to obtain more information about the joint status alterations making the decision on management easier.

Panoramic radiography is probably the most frequently used method as a supplement to the clinical examination of patients with TMD because of its availability. However, the reliability of this method for the diagnostic assessment of the mandibular condyle, which is the only component of the joint that can be examined with this method, is low because it reveals only gross changes and is subject to image distortion. Thus, if one suspects TMJ pathology and the panoramic view is equivocal, CBCT or CT should be considered.

REFERENCES

1. Schiffman E, Ohrbach R, Truelove E, et al. Diagnostic criteria for temporomandibular disorders (DC/TMD) for clinical and research applications: recommendations of the international RDC/TMD consortium network* and orofacial pain special interest group†. J Oral Facial Pain Headache 2014;28(1): 6–27.
2. Annandale T. On displacement of the inter-articular cartilage of the lower jaw, and its treatment by operation. Lancet 1887;129(3313):411.
3. Larheim TA. Current trends in temporomandibular joint imaging. Oral Surg Oral Med Oral Pathol Oral Radiol Endod 1995;80(5):555–76.
4. Farrar WB, McCarty WL Jr. Inferior joint space arthrography and characteristics of condylar paths in internal derangements of the TMJ. J Prosthet Dent 1979;41(5):548–55.
5. Kircos LT, Ortendahl DA, Mark AS, et al. Magnetic resonance imaging of the TMJ disc in asymptomatic volunteers. J Oral Maxillofac Surg 1987;45(10):852–4.
6. Katzberg RW, Westesson PL, Tallents RH, et al. Anatomic disorders of the temporomandibular joint disc in asymptomatic subjects. J Oral Maxillofac Surg 1996;54(2):147–53 [discussion 153–5].
7. Larheim TA, Westesson P, Sano T. Temporomandibular joint disk displacement: comparison in asymptomatic volunteers and patients. Radiology 2001; 218(2):428–32.
8. Turp JC, Schlenker A, Schroder J, et al. Disk displacement, eccentric condylar position, osteoarthrosis - misnomers for variations of normality? Results and interpretations from an MRI study in two age cohorts. BMC Oral Health 2016;16(1):124.
9. Westesson PL, Eriksson L, Kurita K. Reliability of a negative clinical temporomandibular joint examination: prevalence of disk displacement in asymptomatic temporomandibular joints. Oral Surg Oral Med Oral Pathol 1989;68(5):551–4.
10. Tasaki MM, Westesson PL, Isberg AM, et al. Classification and prevalence of temporomandibular joint disk displacement in patients and symptom-free volunteers. Am J Orthod Dentofacial Orthop 1996; 109(3):249–62.
11. Rammelsberg P, Pospiech PR, Jager L, et al. Variability of disk position in asymptomatic volunteers and patients with internal derangements of the TMJ. Oral Surg Oral Med Oral Pathol Oral Radiol Endod 1997;83(3):393–9.
12. Tominaga K, Konoo T, Morimoto Y, et al. Changes in temporomandibular disc position during growth in young Japanese. Dentomaxillofac Radiol 2007; 36(7):397–401.
13. Limchaichana N, Petersson A, Rohlin M. The efficacy of magnetic resonance imaging in the diagnosis of degenerative and inflammatory temporomandibular joint disorders: a systematic literature review. Oral Surg Oral Med Oral Pathol Oral Radiol Endod 2006;102(4):521–36.
14. Westesson PL, Katzberg RW, Tallents RH, et al. Temporomandibular joint: comparison of MR images with cryosectional anatomy. Radiology 1987;164(1): 59–64.
15. Katzberg RW, Westesson PL, Tallents RH, et al. Temporomandibular joint: MR assessment of rotational and sideways disk displacements. Radiology 1988;169(3):741–8.
16. Schwaighofer BW, Tanaka TT, Klein MV, et al. MR imaging of the temporomandibular joint: a cadaver study of the value of coronal images. AJR Am J Roentgenol 1990;154(6):1245–9.
17. Tasaki MM, Westesson PL. Temporomandibular joint: diagnostic accuracy with sagittal and coronal MR imaging. Radiology 1993;186(3):723–9.
18. Musgrave MT, Westesson PL, Tallents RH, et al. Improved magnetic resonance imaging of the temporomandibular joint by oblique scanning planes. Oral Surg Oral Med Oral Pathol 1991; 71(5):525–8.
19. Schmitter M, Kress B, Hahnel S, et al. The effect of quality of temporomandibular joint MR images on interrater agreement. Dentomaxillofac Radiol 2004; 33(4):253–8.
20. Altman DG. Practical statistics for medical research. London: Chapman and Hall; 1991.
21. Nebbe B, Brooks SL, Hatcher D, et al. Magnetic resonance imaging of the temporomandibular joint: interobserver agreement in subjective classification of disk status. Oral Surg Oral Med Oral Pathol Oral Radiol Endod 2000;90(1):102–7.
22. Ahmad M, Hollender L, Anderson Q, et al. Research diagnostic criteria for temporomandibular disorders (RDC/TMD): development of image analysis criteria and examiner reliability for image analysis. Oral Surg Oral Med Oral Pathol Oral Radiol Endod 2009;107(6):844–60.
23. Katzberg RW, Tallents RH. Normal and abnormal temporomandibular joint disc and posterior attachment as depicted by magnetic resonance imaging in symptomatic and asymptomatic subjects. J Oral Maxillofac Surg 2005;63(8):1155–61.

24. Drace JE, Enzmann DR. Defining the normal tempo-romandibular joint: closed-, partially open- and open-mouth MR imaging of asymptomatic subjects. Radiology 1990;177(1):67–71.

25. Morales H, Cornelius R. Imaging approach to temporomandibular joint disorders. Clin Neuroradiol 2016;26(1):5–22.

26. Larheim TA. Role of magnetic resonance imaging in the clinical diagnosis of the temporomandibular joint. Cells Tissues Organs 2005;180(1):6–21.

27. Schiffman EL, Ahmad M, Hollender L, et al. Longitudinal stability of common TMJ structural disorders. J Dent Res 2017;96(3):270–6.

28. Stegenga B, de Bont LG, Boering G, et al. Tissue responses to degenerative changes in the temporomandibular joint: a review. J Oral Maxillofac Surg 1991;49(10):1079–88.

29. Larheim TA, Smith HJ, Aspestrand F. Rheumatic disease of the temporomandibular joint: MR imaging and tomographic manifestations. Radiology 1990; 175(2):527–31.

30. Suenaga S, Nagayama K, Nagasawa T, et al. The usefulness of diagnostic imaging for the assessment of pain symptoms in temporomandibular disorders. Jpn Dent Sci Rev 2016;52(4):93–106.

31. Koh KJ, List T, Petersson A, et al. Relationship between clinical and magnetic resonance imaging diagnoses and findings in degenerative and inflammatory temporomandibular joint diseases: a systematic literature review. J Orofac Pain 2009; 23(2):123–39.

32. Westesson PL, Brooks SL. Temporomandibular joint: relationship between MR evidence of effusion and the presence of pain and disk displacement. AJR Am J Roentgenol 1992;159(3):559–63.

33. Harms SE, Wilk RM, Wolford LM, et al. The temporomandibular joint: magnetic resonance imaging using surface coils. Radiology 1985;157(1):133–6.

34. Manfredini D, Basso D, Arboretti R, et al. Association between magnetic resonance signs of temporomandibular joint effusion and disk displacement. Oral Surg Oral Med Oral Pathol Oral Radiol Endod 2009;107(2):266–71.

35. Rudisch A, Innerhofer K, Bertram S, et al. Magnetic resonance imaging findings of internal derangement and effusion in patients with unilateral temporomandibular joint pain. Oral Surg Oral Med Oral Pathol Oral Radiol Endod 2001;92(5):566–71.

36. Schellhas KP, Wilkes CH. Temporomandibular joint inflammation: comparison of MR fast scanning with T1- and T2-weighted imaging techniques. AJR Am J Roentgenol 1989;153(1):93–8.

37. Lee SH, Yoon HJ. MRI findings of patients with temporomandibular joint internal derangement: before and after performance of arthrocentesis and stabilization splint. J Oral Maxillofac Surg 2009;67(2):314–7.

38. Emshoff R, Brandlmaier I, Gerhard S, et al. Magnetic resonance imaging predictors of temporomandibular joint pain. J Am Dent Assoc 2003; 134(6):705–14.

39. Larheim TA, Katzberg RW, Westesson PL, et al. MR evidence of temporomandibular joint fluid and condyle marrow alterations: occurrence in asymptomatic volunteers and symptomatic patients. Int J Oral Maxillofac Surg 2001;30(2):113–7.

40. Ginalski JM, Landry M, Meuli RA. Normal range of intraarticular fluid in the knee of healthy volunteers: easy evaluation with MRI. Eur Radiol 1993;3(2): 135–7.

41. Larheim TA, Westesson PL, Sano T. MR grading of temporomandibular joint fluid: association with disk displacement categories, condyle marrow abnormalities and pain. Int J Oral Maxillofac Surg 2001; 30(2):104–12.

42. Takahara N, Nakagawa S, Sumikura K, et al. Association of temporomandibular joint pain according to magnetic resonance imaging findings in temporomandibular disorder patients. J Oral Maxillofac Surg 2017;75(9):1848–55.

43. Hasegawa Y, Kakimoto N, Tomita S, et al. Evaluation of the role of splint therapy in the treatment of temporomandibular joint pain on the basis of MRI evidence of altered disc position. J Craniomaxillofac Surg 2017;45(4):455–60.

44. Park HN, Kim KA, Koh KJ. Relationship between pain and effusion on magnetic resonance imaging in temporomandibular disorder patients. Imaging Sci Dent 2014;44(4):293–9.

45. Khawaja SN, Crow H, Mahmoud RF, et al. Is there an association between temporomandibular joint effusion and arthralgia? J Oral Maxillofac Surg 2017; 75(2):268–75.

46. Takano Y, Honda K, Kashima M, et al. Magnetic resonance imaging of the temporomandibular joint: a study of inter- and intraobserver agreement. Oral Radiol 2004;20(2):62–7.

47. Larheim TA, Westesson PL, Hicks DG, et al. Osteonecrosis of the temporomandibular joint: correlation of magnetic resonance imaging and histology. J Oral Maxillofac Surg 1999;57(8):888–98 [discussion: 899].

48. Mitchell DG, Steinberg ME, Dalinka MK, et al. Magnetic resonance imaging of the ischemic hip. Alterations within the osteonecrotic, viable, and reactive zones. Clin Orthop Relat Res 1989;(244): 60–77.

49. Wilkes CH. Internal derangements of the temporomandibular joint. Pathological variations. Arch Otolaryngol Head Neck Surg 1989;115(4):469–77.

50. Schellhas KP, Wilkes CH, Fritts HM, et al. MR of osteochondritis dissecans and avascular necrosis of the mandibular condyle. AJR Am J Roentgenol 1989;152(3):551–60.

51. Larheim TA, Smith HJ, Aspestrand F. Rheumatic disease of temporomandibular joint with development of anterior disk displacement as revealed by magnetic resonance imaging. A case report. Oral Surg Oral Med Oral Pathol 1991;71(2):246–9.

52. Yano K, Sano T, Okano T. A longitudinal study of magnetic resonance (MR) evidence of temporomandibular joint (TMJ) fluid in patients with TMJ disorders. Cranio 2004;22(1):64–71.

53. Zhuo Z, Cai X. Results of radiological follow-up of untreated anterior disc displacement without reduction in adolescents. Br J Oral Maxillofac Surg 2016; 54(2):203–7.

54. Bristela M, Schmid-Schwap M, Eder J, et al. Magnetic resonance imaging of temporomandibular joint with anterior disk dislocation without reposition - long-term results. Clin Oral Investig 2017;21(1): 237–45.

55. Larheim TA, Abrahamsson AK, Kristensen M, et al. Temporomandibular joint diagnostics using CBCT. Dentomaxillofac Radiol 2015;44(1):20140235.

56. Larheim TA, Kolbenstvedt A. High-resolution computed tomography of the osseous temporomandibular joint. Some normal and abnormal appearances. Acta Radiol Diagn (Stockh) 1984;25(6):465–9.

57. Koyama J, Nishiyama H, Hayashi T. Follow-up study of condylar bony changes using helical computed tomography in patients with temporomandibular disorder. Dentomaxillofac Radiol 2007;36(8):472–7.

58. Jacobson JA, Girish G, Jiang Y, et al. Radiographic evaluation of arthritis: degenerative joint disease and variations. Radiology 2008;248(3):737–47.

59. Brooks SL, Westesson PL, Eriksson L, et al. Prevalence of osseous changes in the temporomandibular joint of asymptomatic persons without internal derangement. Oral Surg Oral Med Oral Pathol 1992;73(1):118–22.

60. Ribeiro RF, Tallents RH, Katzberg RW, et al. The prevalence of disc displacement in symptomatic and asymptomatic volunteers aged 6 to 25 years. J Orofac Pain 1997;11(1):37–47.

61. Abrahamsson AK, Kristensen M, Arvidsson LZ, et al. Frequency of temporomandibular joint osteoarthritis and related symptoms in a hand osteoarthritis cohort. Osteoarthritis Cartilage 2017;25(5):654–7.

62. Nakamura T, Matsumoto T, Nishino M, et al. Early magnetic resonance imaging and histologic findings in a model of femoral head necrosis. Clin Orthop Relat Res 1997;(334):68–72.

63. Peck CC, Goulet JP, Lobbezoo F, et al. Expanding the taxonomy of the diagnostic criteria for temporomandibular disorders. J Oral Rehabil 2014;41(1):2–23.

64. Dahlstrom L, Lindvall AM. Assessment of temporomandibular joint disease by panoramic radiography: reliability and validity in relation to tomography. Dentomaxillofac Radiol 1996;25(4):197–201.

65. Crow HC, Parks E, Campbell JH, et al. The utility of panoramic radiography in temporomandibular joint assessment. Dentomaxillofac Radiol 2005;34(2): 91–5.

66. Schmitter M, Gabbert O, Ohlmann B, et al. Assessment of the reliability and validity of panoramic imaging for assessment of mandibular condyle morphology using both MRI and clinical examination as the gold standard. Oral Surg Oral Med Oral Pathol Oral Radiol Endod 2006;102(2):220–4.

67. Brooks SL, Brand JW, Gibbs SJ, et al. Imaging of the temporomandibular joint: a position paper of the American Academy of Oral and Maxillofacial Radiology. Oral Surg Oral Med Oral Pathol Oral Radiol Endod 1997;83(5):609–18.

68. Mercuri LG. Temporomandibular joint disorder management in oral and maxillofacial surgery. J Oral Maxillofac Surg 2017;75(5):927–30.

The Use of Synovial Fluid Analysis for Diagnosis of Temporomandibular Joint Disorders

Gary F. Bouloux, MD, DDS, MDSc, FRACDS, FRACDS (OMS), FACS

KEYWORDS

- Temporomandibular joint • Synovial fluid • Cytokines • Biomarkers

KEY POINTS

- Intra-articular pathologic conditions are associated with qualitative and quantitative changes in multiple synovial fluid biomarkers.
- The biomarkers identified in any given patient may enable a specific diagnosis to be made, including internal derangement, synovitis, chondromalacia, and autoimmune arthritis.
- Biomarkers may be used to monitor disease progression and response to treatment.

INTRODUCTION

Synovial fluid in the temporomandibular joint (TMJ) is a dialysate of plasma that also contains lipids, cholesterol, phospholipids, hyaluronic acid, glycosaminoglycans, albumin, immunoglobulin, elastase, collagenase, cathepsins, proteinase inhibitors, phospholipase A_2, alpha-2-macroglobulin, cytokines, and growth factors, as well as degradation products, inflammatory cells, and mesenchymal stem cells.[1] It provides joint lubrication and stress distribution in addition to providing nutrients and removing waste products of collagen and proteoglycan catabolism.

Synovial fluid is predominantly produced by type B synovial cells that line the nonarticulating surfaces of the TMJ. Various disease states in the TMJ result in alterations in the composition of synovial fluid, including viscosity, hyaluronic acid molecular size, and cytokine levels. Changes in synovial fluid composition provides an opportunity to quantitate and qualitate composition changes in order to potentially diagnose and monitor response to treatment.

The ability to use synovial fluid analysis to diagnose TMJ pathologic conditions is predicated on 3 assumptions:

- Synovial fluid biomarkers should be unique to specific diseases, such as osteoarthritis (OA), autoimmune arthritis, reactive arthritis (ReA), and internal derangement (ID)
- Quantitative biomarker analysis should correlate with disease progression or regression
- Asymptomatic patients without TMJ pathologic condition have a biomarker profile that is different from those with symptoms and/or pathologic conditions

Synovial Fluid and the Healthy Temporomandibular Joint

Synovial fluid sampling from subjects with healthy TMJs has provided much insight into the biological milieu within the TMJ. A healthy TMJ is generally considered to be an asymptomatic TMJ without any radiographic evidence of OA. Synovial fluid from healthy subjects is known to have both

Disclosure Statement: The author has nothing to disclose.
Oral and Maxillofacial Surgery, Emory University, 1365B Clifton Road Northeast, Atlanta, GA 30322, USA
E-mail address: gfboulo@emory.edu

Oral Maxillofacial Surg Clin N Am 30 (2018) 251–256
https://doi.org/10.1016/j.coms.2018.03.001

inflammatory and anti-inflammatory cytokines.[2] The pro-inflammatory cytokines interleukin (IL-2) and tumor necrosis factor (TNF) are typically present at low levels, as is the anti-inflammatory cytokine interferon-γ (IFN-γ). Furthermore, the levels of TNF and IFN-γ appear to correlate in healthy subjects, reflecting a balance between inflammatory and anti-inflammatory cytokines in an asymptomatic TMJ.

Synovial Fluid and Temporomandibular Joint Arthropathy

Qualitative and quantitative differences in the cytokine profile between healthy subjects and those with TMJ disease have been previously described.[3–13] A positive correlation between cytokine levels and the presence of disease is generally seen in most studies. Furthermore, many studies suggest that cytokine levels correlate with the extent of the disease. Correlation has been reported for the key cytokines IL-1β, IL-6, IL-11, TNF-α, and transforming growth factor-β1 (TGF-β1).[4–6,9–12,14] These findings would suggest that inflammatory cytokines play a major role in the development and progression of diseases, including ID and OA. Although most studies support these findings, there are some that have failed to show a positive correlation for specific cytokines, including IL-1β,[8,11] IL-6,[15] IL-8,[16] IL-10,[15] and TNF-α.[8,16]

Although the inciting event may differ, the inflammatory response within the TMJ and synovial fluid is similar. Inflammatory arthropathy and ReA are thought to result from activation of the immune system resulting in complement activation and the migration and activation of macrophages and polymorphonuclear leukocytes, and the release of multiple cytokines and growth factors[17] (**Table 1**). Mechanical stress is also thought to result in a similar process, although the mechanism appears to be more complicated. Ultimately, tissue destruction occurs as a result of the generation of free radicals and reactive oxygen species by macrophages and polymorphonuclear leukocytes[18] (**Fig. 1**). The free radicals and reactive oxygen species result in the degradation of proteins and proteoglycans in the synovial fluid, cartilage, bone, and connective tissues. Synovial fluid viscosity is increased, which results in further tissue destruction and impaired lubrication and nutrition of the articular cartilage and disc. The amount of tissue destruction depends on the tissue's ability to scavenge the free radicals and reactive oxygen species (see **Fig. 1**).

Synovial Sampling

Synovial sampling is relatively simple to perform during arthrocentesis and arthroscopy. However, it

Table 1
Cytokine and growth factor content of temporomandibular joint synovial fluid aspirate

Cytokine or Growth Factor	Source	Activity
IL-1α, IL-1β	IC, SC	Pro-inflammatory
IL-1Ra	IC	Anti-inflammatory
IL-2	IC	Pro-inflammatory
IL-4	IC	Pro-inflammatory
IL-6	IC, FB, ET	Pro-inflammatory
IL-6sr	IC	Pro-inflammatory
IL-8	IC, FB, ET, SC	Pro-inflammatory
IL-10	IC	Anti-inflammatory
IL-11	FB, ET, SC	Pro-inflammatory
IL-12	IC	Pro-inflammatory
IL-17	IC	Pro-inflammatory
TNFα	IC	Pro-inflammatory
TNFβ	IC	Pro-inflammatory
sTNFr	Most cells	IR
IFN γ	IC	Pro-inflammatory
TGF-β1	IC	Anabolic, IR
VEGF	Most cells	Angiogenesis
Osteoprotegerin	MSC	Inhibit osteoclasts
TIMP-1	IC	Anti-inflammatory
MMP-3	IC	Pro-inflammatory
MMP-7	IC	Pro-inflammatory
RANKL	Most cells	Bone turnover, IR
ADAMTS	Most cells	Pro-inflammatory

Abbreviations: ET, endothelial cells; FB, fibroblasts; IC, inflammatory cells; IR, immune regulation; RANKL, receptor activator of nuclear factor; SC, synovial cells; sTNFr, soluble tumor necrosis factor receptor; TIMP, tissue inhibitor of metalloproteinases; VEGF, vascular endothelial growth factor.

remains technique sensitive in that it is important to obtain the sample without contamination with blood. Typically, a 1-mL volume of normal saline is injected into the superior joint space using a 22-gauge needle; the mandible is manipulated to ensure the saline and synovial fluid mix, and then the joint fluid is aspirated and sent for analysis. The enzyme-linked immune sorbent assay, polymerase chain reaction (PCR), isobaric tags for relative and absolute quantitation, biotin-labeled-based protein

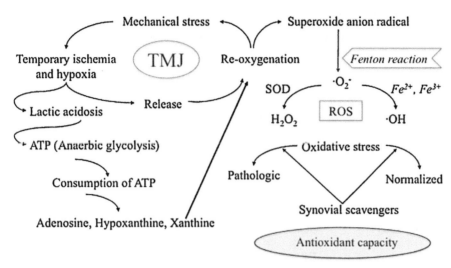

Fig. 1. A common pathway to tissue destruction. ATP, adenosine triphosphate; SOD, superoxide dismutase. (*From* Ishimaru K, Ohba S, Yoshimura H, et al. Antioxidant capacity of synovial fluid in the temporomandibular joint correlated with radiological morphology of temporomandibular disorders. Br J Oral Maxillofac Surg 2015;53:119; with permission.)

arrays, cytotoxic assays, immunostaining, and enzymography have all been used for cytokine assay.[19] The significant differences in the methods used to identify and quantitate cytokines make direct comparisons of results challenging.

Synovial Fluid Composition for Internal Derangements and Osteoarthritis

The pathogenesis of OA in all joints involves aberrations in genetic, biological, and mechanical factors. These aberrations ultimately result in the recruitment of T cells, B cells, and macrophages. Multiple cytokines are released, which initiate and drive an inflammatory response leading to tissue destruction. In addition, metalloproteinases (MMP) and disintegrin and metalloproteinase with thrombospondin motifs (ADAMTS) enzymes are produced, resulting in further degradation of cartilage, bone, synovial proteoglycans, and aggrecan.[20–24]

ID of the TMJ are considered the precursor to OA. The ability to distinguish between the Wilkes stages of ID, including the presence of OA with stages IV and V based purely on cytokine levels or ratios, remains promising. Limitations that currently make this challenging are the following:

- Lack of a large repository of standardized clinical and TMJ cytokine data for healthy TMJs, ID, and OA
- Lack of a simple and standardized technique for synovial fluid sampling
- Lack of consistency in the methods for qualitative and quantitative analysis

However, preliminary data over the last 20 years have provided sufficient evidence to suggest that the cytokine profile for ID and OA are different. Most cytokines are identified in both ID and OA, although the levels and ratios differ. The differences in levels and ratios probably reflects the development of cartilage and osseous degeneration in OA (**Table 2**). The elevated levels of IL-1β, IL-6, IL-6sr, IL-11, TNF-α, sTNFR, and TGF-β1 in OA when compared with ID alone have been reported.[4,5,7–12,14] Il-6 and IL-11 are both thought to induce RANKL expression, resulting in increased osteoclastic activity and in cartilage and osseous destruction. The levels of the anti-inflammatory cytokines IL-10 and OCIF/OPG (Osteoclastogenesis inhibitory factor/Osteoprotegerin) also appear to be reduced in OA. IL-10 plays a key role in inhibiting the synthesis of proinflammatory cytokines, including IL-1α, IL-1β, IL-6, IL-8, IL-12, and TNF-α, as well as stimulating the production of the anti-inflammatory cytokine IL-1RA.[25]

Synovial Fluid Composition in Rheumatoid Arthritis

Consistent differences in serum cytokines and soluble cytokine receptors between rheumatoid arthritis (RA) and juvenile idiopathic arthritis (JIA), as well as between the various subtypes of JIA, have been observed.[26] In RA and JIA, the major site of joint destruction is the pannus, where macrophages and fibroblast-like synoviocytes are present. In response to the abundance of proinflammatory cytokines, these cells produce both MMPs and ADAMTS, resulting in significant tissue destruction. In contrast to OA, Th1 T cells sustain the inflammatory response with the production of IL-2 and IFN-γ.[27]

Table 2
Cytokines found in synovial fluid of patients with internal derangements and osteoarthritis

Author	Cytokines	ID		OA
Fang et al,[4] 1999	IL-1RA	175.78		187.85
	IL-10	ND		ND
	TGF-β1	47.93		143.61
Fu et al,[6] 1995	IL-6	Iliad		—
Fu et al,[5] 1995	TNF-α	3.86		11.27
Kaneyama et al,[8] 2002		*Wilkes I, II*	*Wilkes III*	
	IL-1β	0.14	0.12	0.13
	TNF-α	0.03	0.17	0.17
	IL-6	0.2	14	30
	IL-8	16	13	14
Kaneyama et al,[7] 2003	OCIF/OPG	160		80
	IL-1β	0.08		0.1
	TNF-α	0.4		0.3
Kaneyama et al,[9] 2004	IL-6	5		25
	IL-11	2		7
Kaneyama et al,[10] 2005	IL-1β	0.8		0.6
	IL-RA	42		41
	IL-6	5		5
	IL-6 SR	343		644
	TNF-α	0.1		0.1
	sTNFR	197		261
Shinoda & Takaku,[11] 2000	IL-1β	0.8		1.7
	IL-6	2.1		8.8
	TIMP-I	25.6		120.3
Takahashi et al,[12] 1998		*Wilkes I, II*	*Wilkes III*	
	IL-1β	14.5	7.2	56.9
	IL-6	ND	15.9	7.3
	IL-8	138.1	58.0	50.3
	TNF-α	ND	413	193
	IFN-γ	78.8	36.1	91.8
Wakita et al,[13] 2006		*Wilkes I, II*	*Wilkes III*	
	RANKL	125	100	112.5
	OPG	600	300	200
	RANKL/OPG ratio	0.3	0.4	0.8

An analysis of synovial fluid in RA and JIA suggests that there are several unique characteristics that may provide the opportunity to identify disease as well as monitor the response to treatment. Chronic T-cell activation results in the production of many T-cell-specific cytokines, including IL-2, IL-7, IL-10, IL-12, IL-13, IL-14, IL-15, and IL-17. Although not specific to RA and JIA, TNF-α remains one of the most potent cytokines in RA and JIA, with significantly higher levels. Elevated TNF-α is also the impetus for the development of biologics to block TNF-α in the treatment of these diseases.

Synovial Fluid Composition for Reactive Arthritis

ReA can occur following many bacterial infections; these include *Chlamydia trachomatis*, *Chlamydia pneumoniae*, *Yersinia enterocolitica*, *Campylobacter* species, *Mycoplasma genitalium*, and *Ureaplasma urealyticum*. The inflammatory response in ReA appears to be driven by T cells. The relatively higher proportion of antigen-specific T cells in synovial fluid compared with peripheral blood suggests that the bacteria are sequestered in the joint itself.[28,29] There appears to be a strong correlation between the development of ReA and the presence of the HLA-B27 gene.

The cytokine profile in ReA appears to involve many of the same cytokines seen in RA and JIA. The generation of similar cytokines is the result of the classic Th1 T-cell response that is typical for ReA, RA, and JIA. TNF-α, IFN-γ, and IL-12 are key cytokines in a Th1 T-cell response and are critical for the effective killing of the intracellular pathogens responsible for ReA.[30] Furthermore, it has been suggested that a Th2 T-cell response, which favors a humoral immune response, is associated with the persistence of the bacteria. A predominant Th2 T-cell response is typically associated with elevated levels of IL-10 and reduced levels of TNF-α and IFN-γ. The relative contribution of a Th1 or Th2 T-cell response also appears to be influenced by the antigenicity of the microorganism. There is some evidence that C trachomatis induces a predominantly Th2 T-cell response, which may explain the persistence of the microorganism.[30]

The most sensitive method available to detect the presence of intracellular pathogens remains the PCR, although immunohistochemistry can also be used. The PCR amplifies any bacterial DNA and allows identification of the microorganism. C trachomatis, Mycoplasma fermentans, and Myocoplasma genitalium have all been identified in the TMJ.[31,32] These microorganisms have been shown to reside in the subsynovial tissue within the macrophages and monocytes, necessitating an actual biopsy specimen from the retrodiscal tissue for identification rather than synovial fluid analysis.

The Future

The ability to diagnose the cause of TMJ pain currently relies on a thorough history and physical examination combined with advanced imaging such as MRI. Synovial fluid analysis provides additional information in that the presence of inflammatory mediators and degraded proteins can be identified. The recognition of the same inflammatory mediators and proteins in OA, ReA, and inflammatory arthropathies, despite differing causes, makes it very challenging to identify the specific disease for any given patient using synovial fluid analysis alone.

Proteomics has been suggested as an alternative method to allow a more accurate diagnosis, monitoring of disease activity and severity, and response to treatment.[33] Proteomics is based on the potential for each specific disease to have its own protein profile. Oligoarticular, polyarticular, and systemic JIA can be distinguished based on their differential protein profiles.[34] Patients with OA and those without OA can also be separated based on proteomics even if inflammation is present in both.[35,36] Even more impressive is the ability to distinguish OA from inflammatory arthropathy based on a 3-fold difference in protein level for 135 proteins that have been identified in both diseases.[37]

The potential to make a specific diagnosis with synovial fluid proteomics clearly exists and will in the near future enable the clinician to make a diagnosis with great sensitivity and specificity as well as monitor disease progression and response to treatment.

REFERENCES

1. Bouloux GF. Temporomandibular joint pain and synovial fluid analysis: a review of the literature. J Oral Maxillofac Surg 2009;67:2497–504.
2. Kristensen KD, Alstergren P, Stoustrup P, et al. Cytokines in healthy temporomandibular joint synovial fluid. J Oral Rehabil 2014;41:250–6.
3. Jiang Q, Qiu YT, Chen MJ, et al. Synovial TGF-beta1 and MMP-3 levels and their correlation with the progression of temporomandibular joint osteoarthritis combined with disc displacement: a preliminary study. Biomed Rep 2013;1:218–22.
4. Fang PK, Ma XC, Ma DL, et al. Determination of interleukin-1 receptor antagonist, interleukin-10, and transforming growth factor-beta1 in synovial fluid aspirates of patients with temporomandibular disorders. J Oral Maxillofac Surg 1999;57:922–8 [discussion: 928–9].
5. Fu K, Ma X, Zhang Z, et al. Tumor necrosis factor in synovial fluid of patients with temporomandibular disorders. J Oral Maxillofac Surg 1995;53:424–6.
6. Fu K, Ma X, Zhang Z, et al. Interleukin-6 in synovial fluid and HLA-DR expression in synovium from patients with temporomandibular disorders. J Orofac Pain 1995;9:131–7.
7. Kaneyama K, Segami N, Nishimura M, et al. Osteoclastogenesis inhibitory factor/osteoprotegerin in synovial fluid from patients with temporomandibular disorders. Int J Oral Maxillofac Surg 2003;32:404–7.
8. Kaneyama K, Segami N, Nishimura M, et al. Importance of proinflammatory cytokines in synovial fluid from 121 joints with temporomandibular disorders. Br J Oral Maxillofac Surg 2002;40:418–23.
9. Kaneyama K, Segami N, Sato J, et al. Interleukin-6 family of cytokines as biochemical markers of osseous changes in the temporomandibular joint disorders. Br J Oral Maxillofac Surg 2004; 42:246–50.
10. Kaneyama K, Segami N, Sun W, et al. Analysis of tumor necrosis factor-alpha, interleukin-6, interleukin-1beta, soluble tumor necrosis factor receptors I and II, interleukin-6 soluble receptor, interleukin-1 soluble receptor type II, interleukin-1 receptor antagonist, and protein in the synovial fluid of patients with temporomandibular joint disorders. Oral Surg Oral Med Oral Pathol Oral Radiol Endod 2005;99:276–84.
11. Shinoda C, Takaku S. Interleukin-1 beta, interleukin-6, and tissue inhibitor of metalloproteinase-1 in the synovial fluid of the temporomandibular joint with respect to cartilage destruction. Oral Dis 2000;6: 383–90.

12. Takahashi T, Kondoh T, Fukuda M, et al. Proinflammatory cytokines detectable in synovial fluids from patients with temporomandibular disorders. Oral Surg Oral Med Oral Pathol Oral Radiol Endod 1998;85:135–41.

13. Wakita T, Mogi M, Kurita K, et al. Increase in RANKL: OPG ratio in synovia of patients with temporomandibular joint disorder. J Dent Res 2006;85:627–32.

14. Kubota E, Kubota T, Matsumoto J, et al. Synovial fluid cytokines and proteinases as markers of temporomandibular joint disease. J Oral Maxillofac Surg 1998;56:192–8.

15. Vernal R, Velasquez E, Gamonal J, et al. Expression of proinflammatory cytokines in osteoarthritis of the temporomandibular joint. Arch Oral Biol 2008;53:910–5.

16. Wake M, Hamada Y, Kumagai K, et al. Up-regulation of interleukin-6 and vascular endothelial growth factor-A in the synovial fluid of temporomandibular joints affected by synovial chondromatosis. Br J Oral Maxillofac Surg 2013;51:164–9.

17. Akdis M, Burgler S, Crameri R, et al. Interleukins, from 1 to 37, and interferon-gamma: receptors, functions, and roles in diseases. J Allergy Clin Immunol 2011;127:701–21.e1-70.

18. Ishimaru K, Ohba S, Yoshimura H, et al. Antioxidant capacity of synovial fluid in the temporomandibular joint correlated with radiological morphology of temporomandibular disorders. Br J Oral Maxillofac Surg 2015;53:114–20.

19. Kellesarian SV, Al-Kheraif AA, Vohra F, et al. Cytokine profile in the synovial fluid of patients with temporomandibular joint disorders: a systematic review. Cytokine 2016;77:98–106.

20. Malemud CJ. Biologic basis of osteoarthritis: state of the evidence. Curr Opin Rheumatol 2015;27:289–94.

21. Meszaros E, Malemud CJ. Prospects for treating osteoarthritis: enzyme-protein interactions regulating matrix metalloproteinase activity. Ther Adv Chronic Dis 2012;3:219–29.

22. Gargiulo S, Gamba P, Poli G, et al. Metalloproteinases and metalloproteinase inhibitors in age-related diseases. Curr Pharm Des 2014;20:2993–3018.

23. Verma P, Dalal K. ADAMTS-4 and ADAMTS-5: key enzymes in osteoarthritis. J Cell Biochem 2011;112:3507–14.

24. Zhang E, Yan X, Zhang M, et al. Aggrecanases in the human synovial fluid at different stages of osteoarthritis. Clin Rheumatol 2013;32:797–803.

25. de Waal Malefyt R, Abrams J, Bennett B, et al. Interleukin 10 (IL-10) inhibits cytokine synthesis by human monocytes: an autoregulatory role of IL-10 produced by monocytes. J Exp Med 1991;174:1209–20.

26. Mangge H, Kenzian H, Gallistl S, et al. Serum cytokines in juvenile rheumatoid arthritis. Correlation with conventional inflammation parameters and clinical subtypes. Arthritis Rheum 1995;38:211–20.

27. Smolen JS, Tohidast-Akrad M, Gal A, et al. The role of T-lymphocytes and cytokines in rheumatoid arthritis. Scand J Rheumatol 1996;25:1–4.

28. Sieper J, Braun J, Wu P, et al. T cells are responsible for the enhanced synovial cellular immune response to triggering antigen in reactive arthritis. Clin Exp Immunol 1993;91:96–102.

29. Fendler C, Wu P, Eggens U, et al. Longitudinal investigation of bacterium-specific synovial lymphocyte proliferation in reactive arthritis and lyme arthritis. Br J Rheumatol 1998;37:784–8.

30. Braun J, Sieper J. Cytokines and the immunopathology of the spondyloarthropathies. Curr Rheumatol Rep 1999;1:67–77.

31. Henry CH, Hudson AP, Gerard HC, et al. Identification of Chlamydia trachomatis in the human temporomandibular joint. J Oral Maxillofac Surg 1999;57:683–8 [discussion: 689].

32. Henry CH, Hughes CV, Gerard HC, et al. Reactive arthritis: preliminary microbiologic analysis of the human temporomandibular joint. J Oral Maxillofac Surg 2000;58:1137–42 [discussion: 1143–4].

33. Park YJ, Chung MK, Hwang D, et al. Proteomics in rheumatoid arthritis research. Immune Netw 2015;15:177–85.

34. Rosenkranz ME, Wilson DC, Marinov AD, et al. Synovial fluid proteins differentiate between the subtypes of juvenile idiopathic arthritis. Arthritis Rheum 2010;62:1813–23.

35. Pan X, Huang L, Chen J, et al. Analysis of synovial fluid in knee joint of osteoarthritis: 5 proteome patterns of joint inflammation based on matrix-assisted laser desorption/ionization time-of-flight mass spectrometry. Int Orthop 2012;36:57–64.

36. Hsueh MF, Onnerfjord P, Kraus VB. Biomarkers and proteomic analysis of osteoarthritis. Matrix Biol 2014;39:56–66.

37. Balakrishnan L, Bhattacharjee M, Ahmad S, et al. Differential proteomic analysis of synovial fluid from rheumatoid arthritis and osteoarthritis patients. Clin Proteomics 2014;11:1.

Occlusal Equilibration for the Management of Temporomandibular Disorders

Daniele Manfredini, DDS, MSc, PhD*

KEYWORDS

- Temporomandibular disorders • Occlusal equilibration • Occlusal adjustment
- Temporomandibular joint • Gnathology

KEY POINTS

- Historically, the focus of dental professionals approaching patients with temporomandibular disorders (TMDs) has been solely based on the assessment and correction of purported abnormalities of the occlusion.
- The so-called myths of gnathology have been dismantled by the increasing knowledge of the masticatory system and the factors that determine the onset of signs and/or symptoms in the temporomandibular joint or jaw muscles.
- For altered occlusion to be a clinical factor in the diagnosis and management of TMDs, a cause-and-effect relationship should exist between the 2 conditions, but the literature does not support such a relationship.
- Studies on the use of occlusal equilibration to manage TMDs do not support its usefulness.
- Protocols for occlusal equilibration are not backed up with any solid biological background.

INTRODUCTION

The group of conditions collectively included under the umbrella term "temporomandibular disorders" (TMDs) has historically been related to altered dental occlusion ever since the otolaryngologist James Costen, in the first half of last century, described otherwise unexplainable symptoms around the preauricular area of some individuals without molar support.[1] The absence of a full dentition was hypothesized as the source of posterior condylar displacement in the temporomandibular joint (TMJ), with subsequent symptom onset due to compression of the retrodiscal and ear structures. From that time on, dentists have been periodically invoking altered dental occlusion as being the cause of TMDs.

A quick overview of Costen's work shows that he merely used a series of cases in support of his hypothesis.[1] Moreover, one must wonder if the loss of molar support was so rare in the 1930s as to be a discriminator for identifying individuals with clinical consequences. Notwithstanding, the impact of Costen's work was of paramount importance in the history of TMD practice. Apart from giving his name to the disease (ie, Costen syndrome), his most notable contribution involved identification of the dentist as the primary caregiver for conditions that, based on current knowledge, have little or nothing to do with the absence of teeth or the presence of purported malocclusions.[2,3] However, it is because of such work that for years the focus of dental professionals approaching patients with TMDs has been solely based on the assessment and correction of purported abnormalities of the occlusion.[4]

Disclosure: The author has nothing to disclose.
Department of Medical Biotechnologies, School of Dental Medicine, University of Siena, Strada delle Scotte 4, 53100 Siena, Italy
* Via Ingolstadt 3, Marina di Carrara (MS) 54033, Italy.
E-mail address: daniele.manfredini@tin.it

Oral Maxillofacial Surg Clin N Am 30 (2018) 257–264
https://doi.org/10.1016/j.coms.2018.04.002
1042-3699/18/© 2018 Elsevier Inc. All rights reserved.

Over the past few decades, emerging evidence has grown in support of a biopsychosocial model of TMD pain.[5] Notwithstanding, it seems that the new paradigm linking TMD more to central than occlusal/anatomic factors has not been fully accepted by some clinicians. The difficulty in integrating it within the armamentarium of professional skills has a historical (eg, primary role of the dentist as the caregiver for TMD patients), a social (eg, financial disincentives associated with the reduced importance of dental occlusion; patients' expectations), and a clinical (eg, paradox effects of occlusion-oriented therapies such as oral appliances) background. The gap between research and practice can be easily perceived by browsing the Internet and looking at the number of congresses, events, and technological devices that still focus on the search for an ideal occlusion in "dysfunctional" patients. Fancy theories on the relationship between body posture and occlusal abnormalities, which have been dismantled by all reviews on the topic, clearly exemplify the situation.[6,7]

Based on these premises, the present discussion reviews the concept of using occlusal equilibration for the purpose of TMD management based on an overview of the available literature within the context of the historical background and current treatment concepts.

HISTORICAL BACKGROUND

The concept of equilibrating the occlusion to treat and/or to prevent TMDs found its background in the old precepts of gnathology. Gnathology, referred to as the science that studies the function of the organ of mastication, has historically been pursuing the holy grail of an ideal dental occlusion.[8] The fascinating issue of the relationship between form and function, with the latter deriving from the former, has permeated all dental specialties. Orthodontists referred to "mal"occlusions to indicate all dental occlusions that deviates from the ideal,[9,10] and prosthodontists coined the term "centric relation (CR)" to indicate the ideal condylar position in the glenoid fossa.[11] The derivative "centric occlusion" was thus assumed as an ideal position of maximum intercuspation (MI) in CR, and was considered a needed criterion for the absence of masticatory dysfunction and in planning treatment of the dental occlusion.[12] During the mechanistic era of orthodontic gnathology, several techniques and devices were proposed as an aid for the clinician in creating a purported harmony between form and function.

Year after year, the fallacies of the gnathological dogmas have progressively emerged. In addition, the absence of an ideal occlusion-to-TMJ relationship in nature was recognized, and criticism grew against possible overestimation of the importance of such diverse occlusions in the development of TMJ dysfunction. Clinical research has shifted the horizon of TMD pain assessment toward the psychological sphere, and empirical observations of TMD symptom improvement after occlusal equilibration have received alternative explanations.[13]

The so-called myths of gnathology have been dismantled by the increasing knowledge about the masticatory system and the factors that determine the onset of signs and/or symptoms within the TMJ or jaw muscles. In particular, those early theories suggesting that an imperfect occlusion and condylar position are the primary cause of TMDs, and implicitly implying that TMD treatment should be based on the principles of gnathology and occlusal equilibration, have never been supported by solid proof.[14] Nevertheless, the proponents of occlusion-oriented views of TMD treatment keep on producing anecdotes, expressing opinions, and writing letters to journal editors to feed what seems to be a clash of cultures.[15–17]

The missing point in these claims is that for an altered occlusion to be a factor in the diagnosis and management of TMDs, a cause-and-effect relationship should exist between the 2 conditions,[18] which means that among the several criteria that must be satisfied to support any causality claims, the presence of a strong and consistent association between certain occlusal features and TMDs is a basic requirement. Even the disappearance or decrease of symptoms after occlusal equilibration in a single individual is a clinical phenomenon that may have various interpretations depending on the epidemiology of the occlusion-TMD association as well as the pathophysiology of the TMD pain.[5–19] Within this premise, the literature on the association between TMDs and altered dental occlusion, as well the effects of occlusal equilibration in the management of TMDs, are reviewed and discussed in the following sections.

ARE CERTAIN FEATURES OF DENTAL OCCLUSION ASSOCIATED WITH TEMPOROMANDIBULAR DISORDERS?

In the science of medical epidemiology, an association between 2 phenomena is considered *strong* when they are more frequently present or absent concurrently than singularly. In other words, a certain occlusal feature should be more frequently present in TMD patients than in healthy individuals, and more frequently absent in healthy individuals than in TMD patients. Such an association is *consistent* when confirmed by most research. As previously stated, an association does not mean causality, and the demonstration of an association is only the first criterion to consider as the basis for a possible cause-and-effect relationship between the 2 conditions.

A recent literature review provides a qualitative answer to the very basic clinical research question: "Is there any association between features of the occlusion and temporomandibular disorders?"[3] The findings show a general absence of a clinically relevant association between TMDs and dental occlusion. Among the almost 40 singularly or combined occlusal features that have been assessed in the 25 papers that passed filters for inclusion in the review, only 2 (ie, CR-MI slide and mediotrusive interferences) were associated with TMDs in the majority (ie, at least 50%) of single variable analyses in patient populations. Only mediotrusive interferences were associated with TMDs in most of the multiple variable analyses, with an odds ratio of 2.45 for myofascial pain[20] and 2.14 for disc displacement.[21] Other potential clinically relevant odds ratios for TMDs (ie, higher than 2) in multiple variable analysis have been reported only occasionally.

As a general remark, it can be concluded that features of static occlusion, such as crossbite, deep bite, and dental class, have little or nothing to do with the presence of TMDs.[3] To cite a few findings from studies on patient populations, deep bite was not associated with TMD in any of the 10 studies; large overjet was only noted in one of 8 studies that reported an association with TMJ pain[22]; open bite was noted in one of 8 studies that reported an association with primary osteoarthrosis[23]; and unilateral crossbite was mentioned in only 2 of 6 studies, both performed on the very same population and reporting an association with intracapsular TMJ disorders.[23,24] Thus, the absence of the fundamental prerequisite of an association between the 2 phenomena leads to the conclusion that a causal role for static dental occlusion in TMDs should not be hypothesized.

These findings provide an epidemiologic background to explain observations from a comprehensive clinical study on more than 600 patients, which reported that the correction of orthodontic "malocclusions" is not effective in treating TMDs and that non correction or even imperfect correction are not a cause of TMDs at the population level.[25] As a consequent clinical recommendation, it is now clear that working on tooth alignment within the framework of pursuing an ideal occlusion to improve TMD symptoms is, at best, neutral, namely, it neither treats nor causes TMDs.[25-27]

Moreover, it should be noted that, despite the fact that the dental literature has predominantly been directed toward the view of occlusion as the cause of TMDs, the inverse relationship should also have been considered. That is, the occasionally described associations might even be because of the presence of occlusal features that are secondary to the TMDs. A typical example is the relationship between an anterior open bite and TMJ osteoarthrosis, with the former being the consequence rather than the cause of the latter.[28,29] In addition, the association between unilateral crossbite and TMDs, which was described in 3 of the reviewed studies, has been recently shown to be independent of its correction,[30] which means that in patients with TMDs, the presence of a crossbite is not causative of joint pathologic condition, but rather it can be viewed as the consequence of a certain skeletal morphology, as happens in the case of sagittal skeletal profiles, which are associated with an increased risk for disc displacement.[31]

OCCLUSAL EQUILIBRATION FOR TREATING TEMPOROMANDIBULAR DISORDERS

Although the previously reviewed literature is conclusive regarding the lack of an association between TMDs and features of static dental occlusion, it leaves the door open for a discussion regarding the functional occlusion. The concept that a discrepancy between the ideal pattern of mouth closure in CR and MI leads to orthopedic instability and subsequent joint disorders is a heritage of gnathological principles and is supported by only a few studies reporting a higher prevalence of CR-MI slides and functional interferences in TMD patients.[20-22] The possible existence of some premature tooth contacts that shift the mandible from CR to MI, or that interfere with lateral and/or protrusive excursions, has led to the proposal of several strategies to adjust the dental occlusion in TMD patients.[32-34] This so-called occlusal adjustment, or equilibration, requires selective tooth grinding to achieve the best possible fit between the 2 positions. Proponents of such an approach also find support in the empirical observation that oral appliances, which usually cover all the teeth, are effective in relieving pain, thus suggesting an occlusion-mediated mechanism of action.[35] Actually, the available literature has been revisited several times over the past decade, and all reviews suggest that occlusal equilibration to manage TMD symptoms provides questionable effects, without any evidence that it is superior to mock equilibration.[36-39]

With the aim of providing a comprehensive and updated summary of the topic, a systematic literature search in the PubMed and Scopus databases (accessed August 16, 2017), using the key words "temporomandibular disorders" AND "occlusal equilibration" OR "occlusal adjustment" was performed.

A total of 113 hits were retrieved. Titles and abstract screening for the inclusion of articles that actually dealt with occlusal equilibration for the management of TMDs led to the exclusion of 106 references. Thus, 7 articles were read in full text. Search expansion strategies (eg, Medline-related articles, article reference lists, and the author's personal knowledge) allowed inclusion of 3 more articles, for a total of 10 articles. Of those, only 5 were randomized clinical trials (RCTs) comparing occlusal equilibration to other treatment modalities.[40–44] Other studies used a combination of occlusal equilibration and oral appliances in comparison with mock equilibration alone for the management of TMD patients with headache,[45] or in comparison with either counseling or TMJ injections.[46,47] One article reported on an uncontrolled study in which a group of patients with myofascial pain received occlusal adjustment,[48] and another one described a case series of TMD patients treated with mock equilibration alone.[49] Three additional studies, all performed by the same research group, assessed the potential usefulness of real versus mock occlusal equilibration for the prevention, but not the management, of TMDs in adolescents[50,51] or adult women.[52] These 3 studies on the potential benefit of systematically equilibrating the occlusion at 6-month intervals showed it to be superior to mock equilibration for reducing the onset of TMD signs and symptoms over a 3-year follow-up period.[50–52] The risk for TMDs was reportedly to be 8 and 5 times greater, respectively, in adolescents and female adults not undergoing true occlusal adjustment.[51,52] Although these findings are interesting, it should be noted that they lack external validity. A review of the adolescent sample that was assessed meta-analytically showed that the true odds ratio was only slightly in favor of true occlusal adjustment when the preliminary and definitive reports were considered together.[53] In addition, it should be noticed that dropout rates in both the adult and the adolescent samples were much greater in the occlusal adjustment group and that the investigators were not blinded at the follow-up assessments. The fact that there was no information on the psychosocial issues of the participants and that all available data came from the same group of researchers further hampers the generalizability of the findings (ie, external validity). Thus, the evidence either in support or against the use of occlusal equilibration at scheduled intervals to prevent the onset of TMDs is low.

Findings on the use of occlusal equilibration to manage TMDs also do not support its usefulness. Out of the 5 RCTs available in the literature, only one reported a superior effect of interference removal compared with mock elimination.[44] To the contrary, one investigation showed a similar effectiveness with respect to mock equilibration[43]; another 2 reported comparable outcomes with respect to counseling[42] and exercise therapy,[40] and one found an inferiority with respect to a standard conservative protocol providing oral appliances and, when needed, occlusal equilibration.[41]

These results are in line with notable studies showing that mock equilibration alone is enough to achieve the disappearance of symptoms in 64% of patients,[49] and that protocols including adjustment along with an oral appliance are not superior to just counseling or to TMJ injections.[46,47] Taken together, these findings can be considered as supporting the current era of conservative treatment, the understanding of placebo effects, as well as the need for psychological support for TMD pain patients.[54]

DISCUSSION

Based on the previous literature findings, one should consider if there is any rational place for occlusal equilibration in the armamentarium of the TMD practitioner. The first consideration is that most of the available studies date back an average of 30 years, the newest dating back to the late 1990s. Some of them are difficult to appraise based on current knowledge of TMDs and orofacial pain. Standardized clinical guidelines for the evaluation of TMD signs and symptoms were developed after the publication of the early research,[55] but they were never used in later studies. Besides, despite the fact that most studies seemed to focus on patients with myofascial pain, some protocols were unclear about what TMDs were being addressed or, more generally, they involved unspecified TMDs. Relying on nonvalidated measures of dysfunction (eg, Helkimo index) or technological devices with unclear reproducibility (eg, digital occlusal analysis), and arbitrarily giving importance to different signs and symptoms independent of the duration, intensity, and frequency of the pain, are other shortcoming that are difficult to accept. In the end, the absence of any information about the psychosocial impairment of the patients emerges as a factor that may be responsible for randomization bias, based on current evidence that baseline psychosocial impairment is likely the most important predictor of treatment outcome[56] and that treatment-seeking behavior is a crucial factor in discriminating between patient and nonpatient populations with similar physical symptoms.[57]

Notwithstanding, it must be noted that there are some clinical factors that should make occlusal equilibration studies difficult to design and that such shortcomings will inevitably affect any investigations due to the number of empirical clinical variables that can influence the planning and execution of occlusal adjustments at chair side. In particular, the use of the word *equilibration* itself, or adjustment, implies the existence of a predetermined condylar position at the end of the mouth closing pattern or, vice versa, of a dental scheme that eases jaw excursions.

Based on occlusal equilibration theories, any minor obstacle, in the form of either premature contacts during occlusion (eg, CR-MI slide) or disocclusion (eg, mediotrusive, laterotrusive, protrusive interferences), that deviates the mandible from the ideal trajectory of movement should be removed. Standardizing such adjustment, which requires an iatrogenic grinding of teeth to increase interarch fitting in CR or to enhance guidance during excursions, relies on some dogmas that are clinically questionable. For instance, it implies a concurrent standardization of CR recording procedures. Unfortunately, current evidence suggests that CR recordings are inherently biased by the preconceived ideas underlying any specific procedures.[58] That is, manually induced positions, such as those achieved by mandible manipulation, are hardly comparable to artificially induced positions obtained by the use of technological devices or the so-called deprogramming appliances. To put this concept into a clinical framework, this means that the same patient would receive different types of adjustment based on the CR recording procedure, and that the amount of equilibration would be greater the more artificially induced the position.

This uncertainty is further supported by studies showing an absence of imaging-detected differences between condylar positions in CR and MI,[59] thus questioning the generalizability of the concept of orthopedic instability itself when minor occlusal shifts are present. Moreover, in TMD patients, motor adaptation to pain or fatigue can alter jaw movements as well as the instrumental signs that are purportedly associated[60–62] so that the clinician might be induced into a cognitive error.[63] An example of such an error is that a CR-MI slide is interpreted as the cause of TMD pain because of the occlusion-oriented model of disease the clinician is applying. If a correct neurophysiologic interpretation of the findings is applied, a CR-MI slide could be the consequence and not the cause of muscle pain. The latter interpretation fits with sports medicine observations of unsteady and less repeatable joint excursions when agonist muscles are fatigued[64,65] and, more importantly, with current evidence supporting a causal role for prolonged muscle tension exerted via jaw clenching in the cause of TMD pain.[66] Based on these factors, it seems reasonable to conclude that protocols of occlusal equilibration are not supported by any solid biological background or analogy with other musculoskeletal regions.

In addition to any consideration of the doubtful effectiveness and technical uncertainty in execution, it must also be borne in mind that occlusal equilibration requires removal of a certain amount of tooth substance. Such a procedure, even if minimal, is irreversible. Also, enhancement of tooth sensitivity due to concurrent sleep bruxism, as well as of occlusal hypervigilance due to neurologic phenomena such as occlusal dysesthesia, exemplifies the uncertain risk-to-benefit ratio of any occlusal equilibration. The fact that such procedures need to be repeated on a scheduled basis, as per protocols described by the proponents,[48,52] further limits their sustainability in terms of cost and risks of overtreating patients.

The previous findings tend to exclude any use of equilibration at the general population level, but one has to consider if there is some potential benefit at the individual level. Current knowledge does not provide any information about the actual efficacy with respect to subjective effectiveness potentially related to occlusion-unrelated factors (eg, placebo effects; patient expectations; clinician's empathy; treatment of nonrelevant symptoms; or favorable natural course of the disease). Thus, the overuse of any irreversible occlusal procedure based on empirical and anecdotal evidence cannot be supported from an ethical viewpoint based on the financial, biological, and psychological considerations.[67,68] Ideally, proponents of such procedures need to prove validity before claiming any need for altering the occlusion as part of the management protocol for TMD patients. The current state-of-the-art supports the usefulness of conservative approaches, and it is the duty of those practicing outside of these boundaries to prove anything different.

Future studies on healthy volunteers assessing the repeatability of any occlusal recording procedures are the starting point for gathering normal data that should be used as a baseline for comparison with TMD patients. Within this framework, it is also notable that iatrogenic changes of the occlusion are almost an inevitable occurrence during an individual's lifespan and should be considered one of the reasons for the difficulty in assessing the need for adjusting interarch relationships. Moreover, recent suggestions that even unsuccessful orthodontics, namely, not providing an ideal occlusal relationship at the end of treatment, does not increase the risk for TMDs,[25] is an indirect confirmation of the very extensive accommodation skills of the stomatognathic system.

Possible further research on dental occlusion could involve bruxism-related investigations. For example, the effects of prolonged clenching in individuals with an unsteady dental occlusion is worthy of exploration. On the other hand, it must be noted that the bruxism-TMD relationship seems to be independent of the occlusal pattern.[69,70] At worst, jaw clenching in individuals with extreme malocclusions (ie, anterior open bite and large overjet) seems to be associated with a greater frequency of TMJ disorders than with myofascial pain problems. Based on that, patients with occlusal hypervigilance and teeth contacting habit behaviors should be approached with behavioral strategies, instead of focusing on correction of dental occlusion as a purported strategy to make them stop the behavior.[61]

Finally, analogies to using occlusal adjustment for treating TMDs are not biologically plausible for other joints. Possible examples of irreversibly adjusting the endpoint of movement to treat symptoms of the knee, shoulder, or ankle joints, just to cite a few, are scenarios that are difficult to imagine and should be taken into consideration when contemplating such an approach for the TMJ. Thus, it is difficult to imagine that future investigations will dismantle current beliefs that caution clinicians against the use of irreversible occlusal equilibration for the treatment of TMDs.

SUMMARY

There are few reports supporting the effectiveness of occlusal equilibration for treating TMDs. Such reports are mainly outdated studies, case reports, and anecdotal information. Given the irreversible nature of such an approach, and the unfavorable biological and financial cost-to-benefit ratios, the use of occlusal equilibration for TMD management is not recommended.

REFERENCES

1. Costen JB. A syndrome of ear and sinus symptoms dependent upon disturbed function of the temporomandibular joint. Ann Otol Rhinol Laryngol 1934;43:1–15.

2. Okeson JP. Evolution of occlusion and temporomandibular disorder in orthodontics: past, present, and future. Am J Orthod Dentofacial Orthop 2015;147(5 suppl):S216–23.

3. Manfredini D, Lombardo L, Siciliani G. Temporomandibular disorders and dental occlusion. A systematic review of association studies: end of an era? J Oral Rehabil 2017;44(11):908–23.

4. Türp JC, Greene CS, Strub JR. Dental occlusion: a critical reflection on past, present and future concepts. J Oral Rehabil 2008;35:446–53.

5. Suvinen TI, Kemppainen P, Könönen M, et al. Review of aetiological concepts of temporomandibular pain disorders: towards a biopsychosocial model for integration of physical disorder factors with psychological and psychosocial illness impact factors. Eur J Pain 2005;9:613–33.

6. Perinetti G, Contardo L. Posturography as a diagnostic aid in dentistry: a systematic review. J Oral Rehabil 2009;36:922–36.

7. Manfredini D, Castroflorio T, Perinetti G, et al. Dental occlusion, body posture, and temporomandibular disorders: where we are now and where we are heading for. J Oral Rehabil 2012;39:463–71.

8. Kaplan RL. Concepts of occlusion-gnathology as a basis for a concept of occlusion. Dent Clin North Am 1963;7:577–90.

9. Massler M, Frankel JM. Prevalence of malocclusion in children aged 14 to 18 years. Am J Orthod 1951;37:751–68.

10. Emrich RE, Brodie AG, Blayney JR. Prevalence of class 1, class 2, and class 3 malocclusions (angle) in an urban population. An epidemiological study. J Dent Res 1965;44(5):947–53.

11. Moyers RE. Some physiologic considerations of centric and other jaw relations. J Prosthet Dent 1956;6:183–94.

12. Roth RH. Temporomandibular pain-dysfunction and occlusal relationships. Angle Orthod 1973;43:136–53.

13. Laskin DM, Greene CS. Influence of the doctor-patient relationship on placebo therapy for patients with myofascial pain-dysfunction (MPD) syndrome. J Am Dent Assoc 1972;85(4):892–4.

14. Rinchuse DJ, Kandasamy S. Myths of orthodontic gnathology. Am J Orthod Dentofacial Orthop 2009;136(3):322–30.

15. Alanen P. Occlusion and temporomandibular disorders (TMD): still unsolved question? J Dent Res 2002;81:518–9.

16. Slavicek R. Relationship between occlusion and temporomandibular disorders: implications for the gnathologist. Am J Orthod Dentofacial Orthop 2011;139:10, 12, 14 passim.

17. Sutter BA. Phantom bite: a real or a phantom diagnosis? A case report. Gen Dent 2017;65(5):41–6.

18. Hill BA. The environment and disease: association or causation? Proc R Soc Med 1965;58:295–300.

19. Greene CS. The etiology of temporomandibular disorders: implications for treatment. J Orofac Pain 2001;15:93–105.

20. Landi N, Manfredini D, Tognini F, et al. Quantification of the relative risk of multiple occlusal variables for muscle disorders of the stomatognathic system. J Prosthet Dent 2004;92(2):190–5.

21. Chiappe G, Fantoni F, Landi N, et al. Clinical value of 12 occlusal features for the prediction of disc displacement with reduction (RDC/TMD Axis I group IIa). J Oral Rehabil 2009;36(5):322–9.

22. Manfredini D, Peretta R, Guarda-Nardini L, et al. Predictive value of combined clinically diagnosed bruxism and occlusal features for TMJ pain. Cranio 2010;28:105–13.

23. Pullinger AG, Seligman DA, Gornbein JA. A multiple logistic regression analysis of the risk and relative odds of temporomandibular disorders as a function of common occlusal features. J Dent Res 1993; 72(6):968–79.

24. Seligman DA, Pullinger AG. Dental attrition models predicting temporomandibular joint disease or masticatory muscle pain versus asymptomatic controls. J Oral Rehabil 2006;33(11):789–99.

25. Manfredini D, Stellini E, Gracco A, et al. Orthodontics is temporomandibular disorders-neutral. Angle Orthod 2016;89:649–54.

26. McNamara JA Jr. Orthodontic treatment and temporomandibular disorders. Oral Surg Oral Med Oral Pathol Oral Radiol Endod 1997;83(1):107–17.

27. Luther F, Layton S, McDonald F. Orthodontics for treating temporomandibular joint (TMJ) disorders. Cochrane Database Syst Rev 2010;(7): CD006541.

28. Tanaka E, Detamore MS, Mercuri LG. Degenerative disorders of the temporomandibular joint: etiology, diagnosis, and treatment. J Dent Res 2008;87(4): 296–307.

29. Nitzan DW, Palla S. "Closed reduction" principles can manage diverse conditions of temporomandibular joint vertical height loss: from displaced condylar fractures to idiopathic condylar resorption. J Oral Maxillofac Surg 2017;75(6):1163.e1-20.

30. Michelotti A, Iodice G, Piergentili M, et al. Incidence of temporomandibular joint clicking in adolescents with and without unilateral posterior cross-bite: a 10-year follow-up study. J Oral Rehabil 2016;43(1): 16–22.

31. Manfredini D, Segù M, Arveda N, et al. Temporomandibular joint disorders in patients with different facial morphology. A systematic review of the literature. J Oral Maxillofac Surg 2016;74:29–46.

32. Kerstein RB. Current applications of computerized occlusal analysis in dental medicine. Gen Dent 2001;49(5):521–30.

33. Torii K, Chiwata I. Occlusal adjustment using the bite plate-induced occlusal position as a reference position for temporomandibular disorders: a pilot study. Head Face Med 2010;6:5.

34. Solow RA. Clinical protocol for occlusal adjustment: rationale and application. Cranio 2017;1–12. https://doi.org/10.1080/08869634.2017.1312199.

35. Klasser GD, Greene CS. Oral appliances in the management of temporomandibular disorders. Oral Surg Oral Med Oral Pathol Oral Radiol Endod 2009; 107(2):212–23.

36. Tsukiyama Y, Baba K, Clark GT. An evidence-based assessment of occlusal adjustment as a treatment for temporomandibular disorders. J Prosthet Dent 2001;86(1):57–66.

37. Koh H, Robinson PG. Occlusal adjustment for treating and preventing temporomandibular joint disorders. J Oral Rehabil 2004;31(4):287–92.

38. Forssell H, Kalso E. Application of principles of evidence-based medicine to occlusal treatment for temporomandibular disorders: are there lessons to be learned? J Orofac Pain 2004;18(1): 9–22.

39. Weyant RJ. Questional benefit from occlusal adjustment for TMD disorders. J Evid Based Dent Pract 2006;6(2):167–8.

40. Werndal L, Seeman L, Carlsson GE. Occlusal adjustment – mandibular muscle exercise: a comparative study of two methods of treatment of patients with temporomandibular joint pain and dysfunction (in Swedish with English summary). Tandlakartidningen 1971;63:560.

41. Wenneberg B, Nystrom T, Carlsson GE. Occlusal equilibration and other stomatognathic treatment in patients with mandibular dysfunction and headache. J Prosthet Dent 1988;59:478–83.

42. Vallon D, Ekberg EC, Nilner M, et al. Short-term effect of occlusal adjustment on craniomandibular disorders including headaches. Acta Odontol Scand 1991;49:89–96.

43. Tsolka P, Morris RW, Preiskel HW. Occlusal adjustment therapy for craniomandibular disorders: a clinical assessment by a double-blind method. J Prosthet Dent 1992;68:957–64.

44. Kerstein RB, Chapman R, Klein M. A comparison of ICAGD (immediate complete anterior guidance development) to mock ICAGD for symptom reductions in chronic myofascial pain dysfunction patients. Cranio 1997;15(1):21–37.

45. Forssell H, Kirveskari P, Kangasniemi P. Effect of occlusal adjustment on mandibular dysfunction. A double-blind study. Acta Odontol Scand 1986;44: 63–9.

46. Kopp S. Short term evaluation of counselling and occlusal adjustment in patients with mandibular dysfunction involving the temporomandibular joint. J Oral Rehabil 1979;6:101–9.

47. Kopp S, Wenneberg B. Effects of occlusal treatment and intraarticular injections on temporomandibular

joint pain and dysfunction. Acta Odontol Scand 1981;39:87–96.

48. Kerstein RB, Farrell S. Treatment of myofascial pain-dysfunction syndrome with occlusal equilibration. J Prosthet Dent 1990;63:695–700.

49. Goodman P, Greene CS, Laskin DM. Response of patients with myofascial pain-dysfunction syndrome to mock equilibration. J Am Dent Assoc 1976;92: 755–8.

50. Karjalainen M, Le Bell Y, Jämsä T, et al. Prevention of temporomandibular disorder-related signs and symptoms in orthodontically treated adolescents. A 3-year follow-up of a prospective randomized trial. Acta Odontol Scand 1997;55(5):319–24.

51. Kirveskari P, Jamsa T, Alanen P. Occlusal adjustment and the incidence of demand for temporomandibular disorder treatment. J Prosthet Dent 1998; 79(4):433–8.

52. Kirveskari P, Jämsä T. Health risk from occlusal interferences in females. Eur J Orthod 2009;31(5):490–5.

53. Koh H, Robinson PG. Occlusal adjustment for treating and preventing temporomandibular joint disorders. Cochrane Database Syst Rev 2003;(1): CD003812.

54. Greene CS, Goddard G, Macaluso GM, et al. Topical review: placebo responses and therapeutic responses. How are they related? J Orofac Pain 2009;23(2):93–107.

55. Dworkin SF, LeResche L. Research diagnostic criteria for temporomandibular disorders: review, criteria, examinations and specifications, critique. J Craniomandib Disord 1992;6:301–55.

56. Manfredini D, Favero L, Del Giudice A, et al. Axis II psychosocial findings predict effectiveness of TMJ hyaluronic acid injections. Int J Oral Maxillofac Surg 2013;42:364–8.

57. Manfredini D, Ahlberg J, Winocur E, et al. Correlation of RDC/TMD axis I diagnoses and axis II pain-related disability. A multicenter study. Clin Oral Investig 2011;15:749–56.

58. Keshvad A, Winstanley RB. Comparison of the replicability of routinely used centric relation registration techniques. J Prosthodont 2003;12(2):90–101.

59. Lelis ÉR, Guimarães Henriques JC, Tavares M, et al. Cone-beam tomography assessment of the condylar position in asymptomatic and symptomatic young individuals. J Prosthet Dent 2015;114(3):420–5.

60. Lund JP, Donga R, Widmer CG, et al. The pain-adaptation model: a discussion of the relationship between chronic musculoskeletal pain and motor activity. Can J Physiol Pharmacol 1991;69:683–94.

61. Murray GM, Peck CC. Orofacial pain and jaw muscle activity: a new model. J Orofac Pain 2007;21: 263–78.

62. Manfredini D, Cocilovo F, Stellini E, et al. Surface electromyography findings in unilateral myofascial pain patients: comparison of painful vs non painful sides. Pain Med 2013;14:1848–53.

63. Palla S. Cognitive diagnostic errors. J Orofac Pain 2013;27(4):289–90.

64. McMullen KL, Cosby NL, Hertel J, et al. Lower extremity neuromuscular control immediately after fatiguing hip-abduction exercise. J Athl Train 2011; 46(6):607–14.

65. Whyte E, Burke A, White E, et al. A high-intensity, intermittent exercise protocol and dynamic postural control in men and women. J Athl Train 2015;50(4): 392–9.

66. Glaros AG, Marszalek JM, Williams KB. Longitudinal multilevel modeling of facial pain, muscle tension, and stress. J Dent Res 2016;95(4):416–22.

67. Manfredini D, Bucci MB, Montagna F, et al. Temporomandibular disorders assessment: medicolegal considerations in the evidence-based era. J Oral Rehabil 2011;38:101–19.

68. Reid KI, Greene CS. Diagnosis and treatment of temporomandibular disorders: an ethical analysis of current practices. J Oral Rehabil 2013;40:546–61.

69. Manfredini D, Stellini E, Marchese-Ragona R, et al. Are occlusal features associated with different temporomandibular disorder diagnoses in bruxers? Cranio 2014;32(4):283–8.

70. Manfredini D, Vano M, Peretta R, et al. Jaw clenching effects in relation to two extreme occlusal features: patterns of diagnoses in a TMD patient population. Cranio 2014;32(1):45–50.

The Use of Oral Appliances in the Management of Temporomandibular Disorders

Charles S. Greene, DDS[a],*, Harold F. Menchel, DMD[b,c]

KEYWORDS

- Oral appliances • Temporomandibular disorders • Clinical indications • Patient selection

KEY POINTS

- Oral appliances (OAs) can be part of a conservative treatment plan for certain patients with temporomandibular disorders.
- The design of an OA depends on the clinical objectives for each case.
- The mechanisms of action underlying the clinical effects of an OA are not completely understood.
- Using OAs to produce permanent changes in mandibular positions is not supported by current evidence.

INTRODUCTION

There are few topics concerning temporomandibular disorders (TMDs) that elicit more disagreement and controversy than the use of oral appliances (OAs) in treating these disorders. Such devices can be designed to fit in the mouth in several different ways: they can be worn on either the upper or lower arch, they can cover all of the teeth in 1 arch, or they may provide only partial coverage (anterior only, posterior only, covering many teeth or only a few). Their design can be simple (eg, flat occlusal platforms) or they can be modified in several ways: added canine rise ramp, added anterior ramp to force the mandible forward, or added occlusal index to place the mandible in a certain position (eg, centric relation or neuromuscular relationship). They can be prescribed for full-time or part-time wear, and in some protocols they must be worn while eating meals. Some clinicians recommend a specific type of OA for daytime wear and a different type for nocturnal wear, whereas others use upper and lower appliances simultaneously.

Debate also persists regarding how an OA might reduce pain in various components of the stomatognathic system. For example, some clinicians claim that these devices can unload the temporomandibular joint (TMJ); however, it has been shown that this is anatomically impossible even if so-called pivots are added in the posterior areas. However, it may be possible to reduce loading inside the TMJs by a combination of OA design features and specific instructions for usage. Similarly, some clinicians claim that OAs can be used to recapture anteriorly displaced TMJ discs into a normal relationship but others maintain that this is only a temporary success even when it occurs.

The proposition that an OA may reduce the severity of nocturnal bruxism, as well as the amount and intensity of muscular activity at night, has been extensively studied in sleep laboratories. This outcome can occur but it does not occur uniformly in all subjects. For patients with masticatory

[a] Department of Orthodontics (M/C 841), UIC College of Dentistry, 801 South Paulina Street, Room 131, Chicago, IL 60612-7211, USA; [b] Department of Prosthodontics, Nova Southeastern University College of Dental Medicine, 3103-3163 Southwest 76th Avenue, Davie, FL 33314, USA; [c] Private Practice, Coral Springs, FL 33071, USA
* Corresponding author.
E-mail address: cgreene@uic.edu

Oral Maxillofacial Surg Clin N Am 30 (2018) 265–277
https://doi.org/10.1016/j.coms.2018.04.003
1042-3699/18/© 2018 Elsevier Inc. All rights reserved.

muscle pain that seems to be related to nocturnal activities, it has been found that many of them will experience pain reduction from wearing an OA for a few weeks but some will not. For many of the successful patients, the OA can be discontinued without having pain return; but for others that is not possible. These variable outcomes need to be analyzed so that proper clinical decisions can be made.

This article discusses these issues and evidence-based conclusions are provided whenever possible. The main focus is on the use of OAs to treat TMDs; however, there is an overwhelming issue that also needs to be addressed that has not been mentioned yet, namely: What is the ultimate purpose in the mind of a clinician for providing this treatment modality to his or her TMD patient? Clearly, this is a conceptual question with important clinical consequences. At the risk of oversimplification, the authors propose to discuss this issue in terms of the following possibilities:

1. An OA is intended to reduce or eliminate the patient's pain and improve function. It may be used alone or in conjunction with other pain management methods such as medications, physical therapy, stress management, and self-help home care activities.
2. In addition to these goals, an OA is intended to produce a change in the mandibular relationship to the skull, also described as the condyle–fossa relationship. This can occur as a result of muscle relaxation, or it may occur due to specific OA design features. Clinical objectives such as deprogramming and finding optimal mandibular positions are often cited. The new condyle–fossa relationship is generally described as ideal.

In the first concept, there is no irreversible aspect to the use of an OA, and the worst-case outcome potentially should be nothing more than complete failure in the attempt to treat a patient's TMD problem. In the second concept, however, there is an intent to produce an irreversible change in the mandibular position, which later will require an irreversible change in occlusal relationships as well. This treatment concept, which has many different versions within the dental community, is generally referred to as the phase I–phase II approach. Because of the irreversible nature of this approach, a TMD patient could end up with both a failure to improve and a new jaw relationship that is unacceptable. This important clinical controversy is addressed thoroughly in this article.

Controversy 1: Oral Appliance Design: Full Coverage Versus Partial Coverage

The most common design for an OA is a full-coverage device that fits over all the teeth in 1 dental arch, known as a stabilization splint (also described as a Michigan splint). Although some full-coverage OAs are made from inexpensive composite materials that are vacuum-formed in the office, the more classic versions are made from methyl methacrylate acrylic that is processed in a dental laboratory. The latter version requires articulated dental models, a wax-up of the desired design, and careful adjustment of the finished product before it is sent back to the dentist. With the development of thermoplastic inner liners that can be heated with tap water, these devices generally fit quite well over all the teeth and, therefore, usually require little occlusal adjustment. They can be made for either the upper or lower arch, and there is no compelling evidence for preferring either. They should be placed over the arch with the most irregular occlusal plane to ease adjustment and to control thickness. If possible, they should also be placed on the arch with the most posterior teeth to avoid having unopposed teeth that could erupt. In clinical practice, most of these full-coverage OAs are made to cover the maxillary teeth.

There also have been several types of partial-coverage OAs proposed over the years, and various rationales have been offered for choosing to use them. The oldest design is the Hawley anterior biteplate, which is a maxillary appliance that has an occlusal platform from canine to canine. About 40 years ago the mandibular orthopedic repositioning appliance (MORA) was introduced by Gelb and Gelb.[1] This appliance featured a bilateral posterior-only coverage design. The MORA was used by some clinicians to deliberately produce a massive occlusal change in the posterior teeth (**Fig. 1**) that ultimately required major dental restorations on 16 teeth to reestablish the occlusion at a new vertical dimension.

More recently, the idea of a minimal-coverage OA has led to 2 current designs becoming popular. The first is the nociceptive trigeminal inhibition tension suppression system (NTI-tss), which is a commercially available device customized for fit and occlusion in the mouth.[2] A second type is called anterior midpoint stop appliance (AMPSA), which this can be fabricated in the office.[3] Both of these are based on the concept that only 1 to 2 lower anterior teeth should strike the occlusal platform and that this will lead to reflexive relaxation of the masticatory muscles. Many claims have been made about the value of these devices

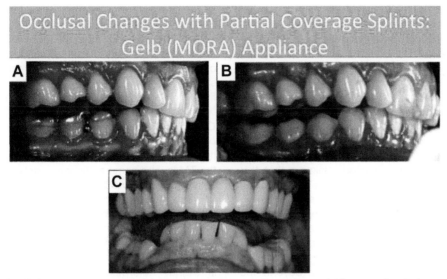

Fig. 1. Occlusal changes in a 24-year-old patient wearing a Gelb appliance 24 hours a day, 7 days a week, for 4 years. (*A*) With appliance in. (*B*) Without appliance. (*C*) Lower occlusal changes in a patient wearing a Gelb MORA appliance for 20 years.

for stopping bruxism, reducing migraine headaches, and eliminating TMD pain.

The main argument for choosing full-coverage versus partial-coverage OAs has been that no dental changes should occur with the former design. Indeed, several types of occlusal changes, including incisor proclination or intrusion, as well as development of an open bite, have been associated with the minianterior devices (**Fig. 2**). The Hawley anterior biteplate, however, covers 6 to 8 anterior teeth and can be quite stable in both the anterior and posterior areas of occlusion as long as strict limitations of only nighttime wear are observed. It has been shown in several electromyography (EMG) and bite force studies that having the posterior teeth out of occlusion will reduce the intensity of muscular activity.[4] Although full-coverage appliances remain the first choice for most patients, they do not prevent tooth clenching, which can be contributing to the myofascial pain, and some patients may keep breaking their appliances. Therefore, in such patients, an anterior biteplate is preferable.

Controversy 2: How Do Oral Appliances Affect Temporomandibular Joint Loading?

In any discussion of OA therapy, it is imperative to have an understanding of the forces acting on the TMJs and how the muscles of mastication create these forces. This understanding is necessary so that the principles of biomechanics can be applied to bite appliance design. Forces on the TMJs have been studied in vivo with animals and humans,[5–8] in vitro,[9–13] with finite element analysis and stereometric MRI, and with joint motion studies.[14] The

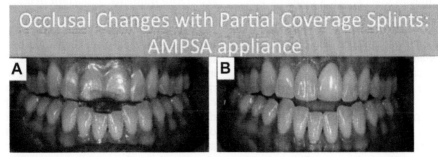

Fig. 2. This appliance was worn for 4 years just at night. (*A*) With appliance in place. (*B*) With appliance out. Notice there is an open bite with contact only on the molars and edge to edge irregularities directly opposing the appliance. The patient reported the change in the lower teeth.

conclusion of all the in vivo studies are consistent in finding that greater posterior tooth contact decreases joint load and that anterior contact increases the load.[15]

Most of the in vitro studies also support this, with few exceptions.[16] There is a consensus in the literature that the TMJ is a loaded joint designed to tolerate normal functional forces of eating, deglutition, and speech.[17,18] There is disagreement about the amount of traumatic or parafunctional force that can be tolerated by the TMJ, with some investigators claiming that this joint is designed to take hundreds of pounds of force.[19,20] However, there is considerable evidence to refute this ridiculous claim; for instance, in vivo clenching forces during arthrocentesis have been measured at only 3 to 4 psi.[6–8] Clearly, not all human TMJs can tolerate the same amount of excessive loading when it goes beyond the physiologic tolerance of the individual.

The areas of contact in the TMJ throughout function are rather broad due to the rotational and translational movements of the joint, and this involves all soft tissues within the joint capsule. The anatomy and structure of the TMJ disc allows for tolerance of higher loads, and the fibrocartilaginous covering of the bony articular surfaces is superior to hyaline cartilage in terms of tissue repair. However, the thinness of the intermediate zone of the disc increases susceptibility to shear forces and creep deformation, with the added possibility of perforations in this area.[21–23] This direct mechanical damage causes the formation of free radicals, further causing other types of joint tissue destruction.[24,25]

Bite force versus joint load

Bite force is determined by elevator muscle contraction. Because the mandible is a class 3 lever system,[26] the more posterior the tooth contact the more bite force that can be generated, whereas the joint load will be reduced. When the posterior teeth are in solid occlusal contact, they absorb the force of muscle contraction. If posterior teeth are missing, or if there is a posterior open bite, then greatly increased bite force is directed to the joints. In patients with anterior disc displacement (ADD), forces are transmitted to the retrodiscal tissues. In some case this will cause pain and inflammation due the vascularity and innervation of this area; however, because this tissue can convert into a fibrous pseudodisc in most ADD patients even if there is no treatment provided,[27] this can enable it to sustain these loads without any pain.

Most studies relating to forces on TMJs use the bite forces generated by the elevator muscles simply because they are easily measured by devices such as EMG or intraoral bite force transducers.[28,29] It is much more difficult to measure actual TMJ loading pressures because to get such measurements requires surgical access, causing tissue damage. Therefore, many of these studies are performed with computer modeling finite element analysis or other indirect means.

Can the temporomandibular joint be unloaded by oral appliances?

It is common to hear or read that an OA can unload the TMJs, and some authorities attribute the success of certain OAs to this feature. However, the concept of unloading the TMJ is often confused with distraction of the joint, which would allow the condyle to move inferiorly and thereby increase joint space. When forces are placed on the TMJ with a normally positioned disc, the disc is slightly deformable and the joint space is decreased.[14] When the forces are reduced, the joint space will return to normal. However, there is no evidence in the literature that any appliance, no matter how it is designed, can unload a TMJ by distraction[30,31] or make any long-term difference in clinical treatment outcomes.[32] However, it is reasonable to consider various possibilities for reducing loading by designing OAs appropriately.

One factor to consider is that a less deformable (harder) material placed between the teeth will stimulate an isometric contraction, as opposed to a more deformable (softer) material that allows for shortening of muscle length. An isotonic contraction generates higher EMG activity, indicating an increased bite force.[33–36] As previously discussed, joint load is reduced when there is posterior support from solid tooth contact or a full coverage appliance. Although bite force is reduced with anterior contacting appliances,[37–40] joint load is increased. Therefore, the dentist can select an appropriate design for each patient based on their different TMD diagnoses and their previous treatment history.

Is anterior guidance important in bite appliance design?

Dentists who routinely place full coverage appliances generally make sure that equal bilateral contacts will occur on full mouth closure. Some also include in their design canine guidance with posterior disocclusion as the mandible moves in lateral excursion. This has been shown in both the natural dentition and with bite appliances to reduce damaging lateral forces to the posterior teeth and implants. Posterior disocclusion also reduces elevator muscle forces, as previously discussed.

What are the effects of posterior tooth contact on the TMJs during bruxism? First, studies have shown that clenching forces, not lateral bruxism, may be paramount factors in the etiology of TMJ degenerative changes.[41,42] Furthermore, in studies with experimental posterior interferences in humans, the joint load is reduced with such tooth contacts.[43] This would be expected considering the previous discussion of joint loading. Owing to a lack of evidence at this time, it cannot be assumed that patients with TMDs will benefit by having their posterior teeth disoccluded during parafunction. Further studies are necessary to determine this.

Controversy 3: How Do Oral Appliances Work to Relieve Temporomandibular Joint Pain?

There are many statements and observations in the dental literature about how OAs may actually work; that is, produce a clinically significant positive treatment outcome. Because so many studies have shown that placebo versions of OAs can produce results that are equal to the real versions, some have questioned whether dentists should even think that OAs are real treatments. As a result of those studies, some investigators have suggested listing OAs as being merely an adjunctive treatment, or even as crutches.[44,45]

However, there are important distinctions that need to be made in discussing this issue. The mixed conclusions reported often are due to the poor experimental design and questionable sampling of many of the OA studies, especially regarding whether the appropriate Research Diagnostic Criteria for TMD (RDC/TMD) diagnoses were used for inclusion or exclusion of the patient sample to be studied. In many studies, there is no differentiation between joint and muscle diagnoses, or between chronic or acute TMDs, leading to conflicting results and conclusions. In addition, some studies have contributed to this confusion by considering TMD as being a single disorder, or by having patients with multiple TMD diagnoses included in a given study.[46]

Although it may be difficult to explain exactly how an OA works to reduce acute muscular TMD pain (although they often are quite successful), it is easier to explain how they help in cases of TMJ pain. There is evidence that there is no difference in the prevalence of bruxism as determined by polysomnography between type I patients and controls as defined by the more recent Diagnostic Criteria for TMD (DC/TMD).[47]

The DC/TMD definitions of myogenous pain (type I) are potentially confusing because they include pain in the jaw, temple, ear, or in front of the ear.[48] The definitions of DC/TMD type II (internal derangements) and type III (pathologic TMJ)

patients are clearer. Therefore, why are many TMD patients with subjective and objective findings suggestive of joint involvement included in the type I categories? Furthermore, MRI studies in type I TMD patients have shown that only 2% who are diagnosed with myogenous pain have no joint problems because disc displacements, bony changes, and joint effusion are common findings (**Table 1**).[49] Given the present evidence base, it seems that TMJ arthralgia and inflammation are common findings in almost all patients with various RDC/TMD diagnoses, even type I. Thus, the percentage of pure muscle pain patients is unknown.

There is sufficient support to show that properly constructed appliances reduce joint load, as previously discussed in the section on TMJ loading. Reducing joint forces can be directly related to reducing pain and further injury to joints, as well as reducing muscle pain and spasm by way of Hilton's law: "The nerve trunk innervating a joint also innervates the motor and sensory component of the muscles that move that joint causing muscle pain and spasm."[50] That many TMD cases involve a combination of muscle and joint pain may help to explain why OAs are helpful to so many TMD patients. It also explains why many EMG studies show reduced muscle activity after joint pain is reduced in TMD patients.[51] In the few studies in which arthrogenous TMD diagnoses were separated, the efficacy of the appliance was significantly better compared with controls, especially

Table 1
MRI findings in research diagnostic criteria for temporomandibular disorder type I versus type II and III subjects

Findings	Myofascial Group RDC/ TMD I	Arthrogenous Group RDC/ TMD II, III
No findings	10%	5%
Disc displacement	63%	85%
Bony changes	68%	58%
Joint fluid	26%	49%
DDWR	34%	50%
DDWOR	11%	15%

Abbreviations: DDWR, disc displacement with reduction; DDWOR, disc displacement without reduction.

MRI findings in patients diagnosed with type I RDC/TMDs diagnoses (myofascial pain with and without limited mouth opening). The percentages do not add up to 100% because there were patients with multiple findings.

From Limchaichana N, Nillson H, Ekberg EC, et al. Clinical diagnoses and MRI findings in patients with TMD pain. J Oral Rehabil 2007;34:237–45; with permission.

over the short-term.[52,53] It has been claimed that there is a better response to appliances in patients who are bruxers; however, this cannot be certain without further studies.

In conclusion, the evidence supports the use of full coverage appliances in TMD patients with arthrogenous pain, with the objective of reducing joint load and inflammation. Simple joint unloading tests can be used during clinical examination to determine if the patient will benefit from appliance therapy. In more complex chronic TMD cases, regardless of the clinical diagnosis, appliance therapy may be of minimal benefit. This is especially true in patients with central sensitization, or with RDC/TMD axis II (psychosocial) considerations. At the very least, appliance therapy needs to be combined with medical, physical, and psychological management in this complex patient population.

Controversy 4: Using Anterior Repositioning Appliances

Another controversy in OA therapy revolves around the routine use of anterior repositioning appliances (ARAs) for management of patients with TMJ and disc disorders (RDC/TMD type II and type III patients). This debate is even more specific when discussing the management of disc displacement with reduction or occasional locking, as defined by Wilkes[54] (Wilkes category II).

ARAs are generally hard acrylic maxillary removable appliances with an anterior ramp that brings the mandible forward into a protrusive position (Fig. 3). The appliance can have a flat occlusal plane, or it may have indentations for the posterior teeth to further retain the mandible in an anterior

position. With an upper anterior ramp design, the lower anterior teeth must be observed for increased mobility and/or sensitivity; however, if the appliance has good posterior support, lower incisor forces can be minimized. Mandibular ARAs have been used but less often. Fixed appliances worn 24 hours a day, 7 days per week (eg, Herbst) have also been used in these patients.[55]

Documented cases of occlusal and even skeletal changes have been reported with continuous use of ARAs, even with only nighttime wear[56]; therefore, patients need to be carefully monitored. There is also recent evidence of condylar remodeling in patients with ARAs and reports of lateral pterygoid myocontracture.[57] Therefore, any decision to use ARAs as part of a treatment plan must take these risks into consideration.

Who might benefit from wearing an anterior repositioning appliance?

Patients with clicking There is no scientific justification for using an ARA in patients with painless clicking of the TMJs and no dysfunction (Fig. 4). It is now known that as many as one-third of the adult general population has asymptomatic ADD that can produce a clicking noise on mouth opening and closing[58]; this phenomenon is described as ADD with reduction (ADDR). It has been reported that about 10% of children ages 6–12 years also have some version of ADDR.[59] It is the overwhelming consensus in the literature that these joint noises often appear and disappear spontaneously, and many longitudinal studies have shown that they do not require any treatment in the absence of pain and dysfunction.[60] The biological basis for this benign outcome is that in most individuals the retrodiscal tissues can readily convert

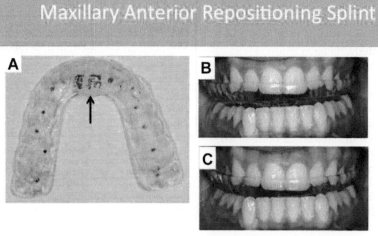

Fig. 3. (A) Full coverage maxillary ARA. With anterior ramp (arrow). Notice the splint is adjusted for posterior support. (B) Splint in place before closure. (C) Complete closure anteriorly repositioning the mandible.

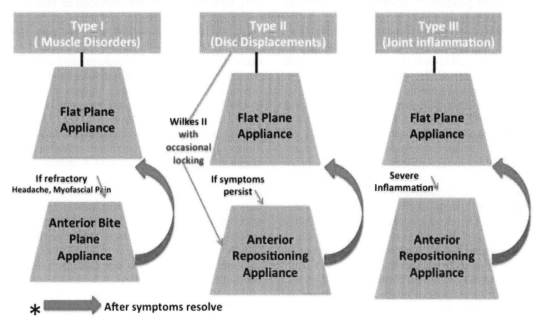

Fig. 4. Flowchart for OA therapy. Type I (myogenous disorders): Patients should have a flat plane appliance as initial therapy. In refractory patients, a trial of an anterior bite plane appliance (eg, Hawley, NTI, AMPSA) is indicated to reduce bite force. When the patient is asymptomatic, return to a flat plane appliance is preferred to avoid any occlusal changes. Note: Anterior bite plane appliances are contraindicated in patients with type II and type III diagnoses. Type II (disc displacements): In patients with no transient locking, a flat plane appliance is the initial therapy. In Wilkes type II patients, initial recommended therapy is an ARA for 2 to 3 months; then return to a flat plane appliance. Type III (TMJ inflammation): Initial therapy is a flat plane appliance. In patients with severe joint inflammation an ARA used for 1 to 2 months, or until inflammation is reduced, may be of benefit; then return to a flat plane appliance.

to become a pseudodisc, which can successfully support condylar loading. This has been demonstrated by postdissection histology and decreased retrodiscal MRI signal from long-standing displaced discs.[61,62]

Although some clinicians have argued for some type of early intervention to avoid future arthritic TMJ problems or joint locking, there is little evidence to support that viewpoint. The concept of prophylactic disc repositioning in patients with painless clicking, which was briefly popular more than 30 years ago, quickly became obsolete because there is no evidence that clicking is a progressive condition in the vast majority of people with ADDR. Likewise, repositioning discs will not prevent degenerative TMJ disease as some practitioners have proposed.[63–65] This concept had been extrapolated from studies of unstable knee injuries that are not treated by surgical ACL repair.[66] These knees do have a higher incidence

of OA but no evidence supports the same pathologic condition occurring in other joints, especially the TMJ. Finally, it should be emphasized that TMJ disc repositioning treatment is also unpredictable (see later discussion).

Of course, patients with painless clicking should be advised that if any pain or transient dysfunction occurs they should be reevaluated and possibly treated. It is also judicious to review the patient's history for any dysfunctional oral habits such as nail biting, gum chewing, or resting on one's hand to support the jaw for extended periods of time,[67] so that appropriate advice can be given.

Patients with painful clicking and arthralgia
Originally it was thought that patients who had painful clicking TMJs should have their discs recaptured and brought back to a correct anatomic position.[68–70] As previously mentioned, failure to do this was believed to lead to

degenerative joint disease, which was thought to be more likely in patients whose clicking had progressed to include pain and dysfunction. ARA therapy to recapture the displaced disc was then often followed with occlusal therapy to maintain the new jaw position. In addition, some type of occlusal procedure usually was required to correct the posterior open bite resulting from long-term ARA wear. It was not very long before the necessity of doing such radical procedures on a routine basis was challenged by several studies in which more conservative approaches were taken.[70–72]

Today it is clear that every disc displacement patient must be evaluated carefully to determine if it is appropriate to place them in an ARA. As stated by Eberhard and colleagues,[73] "The possibility for disc recapture depends on the disc-condyle position and configuration, the integrity of the posterior attachment, and the degree of degenerative change of the intra-articular structures, such as osteophytosis, condylar erosion, or flattening of the articular disc." Recapturing discs was also shown to be more effective in patients with anterior displacement than in those with transverse (sideways) displacement.[74]

Regarding the clinical guidelines for using an ARA, some practitioners advocate only nighttime wear, whereas others advocate full-time wear for as long as 6 months. Some make 2 appliances: 1 for daytime wear and the other for nighttime wear. Some adjust the appliance often, removing acrylic from the anterior ramp to walk the condyle and disc back to a normal position. Others just remove the ramp after a designated period. When this approach fails to produce a successful outcome, surgical procedures to reposition the disc often have been used or recommended.

However, several studies have shown that there were 2 significant problems with this approach. First, the discs that seemed to be clinically recaptured after ARA treatment did not always return to a normal position, nor did they stay there after the appliance was removed.[74] Even if the mandible is stabilized in the protruded position by performing major dental procedures, the discs often slip into a forward position again. Second, it is clear that patients with painful clicking who are treated conservatively can recover without having a disc recapturing procedure and, instead, they can simply resume clicking without having pain or dysfunction. In a recent MRI study, at least 60% of the subjects who had worn an ARA were found to have the disc return to an anterior position after 6 months of therapy; however, most of these subjects are now pain free and have normal mouth opening with no locking, although clicking may have remained.[75] It is likely that longitudinal studies carried out for a longer time would show an even higher percentage of such outcomes.

Another important consideration is that when ADDR patients are given well-adjusted flat plane stabilization appliances with good posterior support, joint noises are often reduced or eliminated passively without anterior repositioning.[76,77] The available studies on ADDR patients who have been treated with flat plane appliances have demonstrated that painful clicking can be reduced by 70% with just these appliances. This positive outcome can also be aided with lysis and lavage of the TMJ, especially when transient locking is part of the clinical symptoms.[78,79]

If there is no history of transient locking, the more conservative approach is to use a flat plane appliance first and then an ARA if necessary.[80] If there is a history of locking, it would be more appropriate to start with an ARA for a limited period. The use of appliances with only anterior tooth contact in patients with disc derangement problems is contraindicated. These have been shown to increase joint noise, possibly due to joint overload.[74] Further in vivo joint loading studies are needed to confirm this.

Patients with temporomandibular joint arthralgia
The presence of pain and inflammation inside the TMJ represents a form of arthritis, by strict definition (RDC/TMD type III). In addition to using other treatment modalities, an ARA might be recommended under certain conditions when stabilization appliances are not effective. For example, a traumatic blow to the mandible might create severe pain and swelling that makes it difficult to close the mouth, similar to what occurs during a severe arthritic flare-up, so positioning the jaw forward for a brief time until the inflammation and pain are reduced could be helpful. A patient who clenches the teeth at night could aggravate his or her joint pain, and a stabilization appliance may not be adequate for treatment of that problem, so there is no harm in positioning this patient's mandible forward for a short period (1–2 weeks) until any joint inflammation has resolved. A person with ADDR or whose disc is no longer capable of reducing might also have a symptomatic flare-up that is best treated for awhile with an ARA because the anterior mandibular position reduces joint loading and will allow healing inside the TMJ.

Controversy 5: How Should Oral Appliances Be Used for Treating Myogenous Temporomandibular Disorders?

The most widely recognized application of OAs for treating TMDs is their use in patients with muscle-related disorders. As previously mentioned, many of these patients may also have TMJ tenderness to palpation but their primary complaints are in the myofascial structures. Most of the controlled clinical trials involving OAs and their placebo counterparts were done with subjects who had a myogenous diagnosis within the RDC/TMD classification. Of these, the most common is myofascial pain, with or without limited mouth opening. In most of these studies, positive results were obtained with both a real OA and a placebo control, but in many studies the real appliance was superior.[81–83] Several systematic reviews and meta-analyses on this topic have been published but unfortunately some of these have included TMD subjects with both muscle and joint diagnoses.[44,84,85] However, an excellent recent review that looked only at myogenous TMD subjects was able to find 8 studies that could be included in their analysis of the effects of a hard stabilization appliance[86] on myogenous pain intensity. Their main conclusion was that there is poor but significant evidence that flat plane occlusal appliances are more effective than nonoccluding appliances when worn during the night only. Other investigators have also offered broad overviews of the application of OAs in treating myogenous pain.[45,87]

An important clinical question is which myogenous TMD patients are likely to be the best candidates for OA therapy. This question is best answered by dividing the population into obvious or suspected bruxism patients versus others (eg, stress-related, traumatic onset, exercise-overload). The bruxism group may have dental wear as evidence of their parafunctional activities, or they may simply report pain and jaw stiffness on awakening, which suggests nocturnal oral activities. These patients are usually excellent candidates for treatment with an OA but a small percentage of them will not respond positively for a variety of reasons, not the least of which is widespread bodily pain as well as chronicity of their pain problem.[88] In such patients, it is commonly found that their pain is associated with depression and sleep disturbance, and that they have 1 or more comorbid conditions such as fibromyalgia, chronic fatigue syndrome, or irritable bowel syndrome.

However, even the successfully treated patients will pose a problem for the clinician; namely, how to conclude the therapeutic relationship. For many of these patients, they can stop using the OA and the pain will not return; this has been demonstrated in several studies and is a very common clinical observation. For those patients whose pain resumes after the OA has been discontinued, there is no reason not to prescribe continued nighttime wear, just as one would for a bruxism patient whose teeth are wearing excessively.

For the types of myogenous TMD pain problems other than myofascial pain, there is no good literature support for using an OA as part of the treatment protocol. The patients who have stress-related problems have been shown to be responsive to a variety of behavioral interventions. For the patient who has had a mandibular block that initiated a myositis problem, the emphasis is on antiinflammatory medications, range-of-motion exercises, heat or cold applications, and possibly physical therapy. For the chronic gum chewer and other oral habit patients, ceasing the habit can be remarkably effective. Lund and colleagues[89] have shown that post-exercise myogenous pain patients may look similar to a bruxism patient, but their problem is acute and situational rather than being continuous, and therefore is not likely to be helped by wearing an OA; the pain-adaptation model of Lund and colleagues[89] has been updated in 2007 by Murray and Peck.[90]

When interviewing and examining TMD patients who seem to have obvious muscular pain problems, the key to proper management is to sort them out according to the diagnostic criteria for myogenous problems as previously mentioned. An especially important issue is whether the pain seems to have a fairly obvious onset pattern and whether it is exacerbated by routine oral functions. These are positive indicators for clinical success in general and, often, an OA can play an important role in their treatment. However, if the pain vaguely arises sometime during the day rather than on waking, varies in intensity for no apparent reason, and is quite diffuse in distribution, the overall prognosis is much poorer, and it is not likely that an OA will make much difference. The patients described by Okeson[91] as having centrally sensitized myofascial pain are the most difficult ones to treat because the chronicity of their pain problem makes it nearly impossible to obtain positive results by using traditional TMD therapies. Therefore, these patients need to be recognized as early as possible so they do not waste time and money in receiving conventional TMD treatments, and they need to be referred for chronic pain management in an appropriate setting.

Controversy 6: Repositioning the Temporomandibular Joint with Oral Appliances

Although all of the previous controversies about OAs are significant, there are even greater ongoing disputes about using them to establish new jaw relationships. These disputes arise from the occlusion and TMJ theories that dominated the twentieth century, in which assumptions were made about the correctness or incorrectness of TMJ positions. In the earliest version of these theories,[92,93] an OA was thought to allow relaxation of the painful masticatory muscles and thereby to reveal occlusal disharmonies, which then could be equilibrated. Other clinicians have recommended using an OA to train or to force the mandible to function in the centric relation (CR) position, which would also require significant occlusal changes to be done afterward. Another version of this thinking is the use of so-called deprogrammer appliances,[94–96] which allow the mandible to be free from occlusal guidance so it can migrate to some "optimal" joint position in which the jaw muscles are relaxed. Finally, there is the neuromuscular version of an OA,[97,98] which is generated by using electronic devices to reduce EMG activity with so-called TENS application. This results in a so-called myocentric jaw position that is usually anterior to other jaw positions.[99] Regrettably, all of these disputes about good and bad jaw positions continue despite the conclusive evidence presented by Rinchuse and Kandasamy (2006) that "the positions of the temporomandibular joint (TMJ) condyles in relation to the glenoid fossa or CR position are not diagnostic of temporomandibular disorders."[100]

All of these interventions can be grouped under a treatment philosophy that is usually described as phase I–phase II therapy, in which an OA is seen as the agent for producing the mandibular position change, and then that change can be stabilized with occlusal modifications. It should be noted that the scope of such occlusal procedures ranges from simple equilibration to orthodontics, full mouth reconstruction, bite opening, and even orthognathic surgery. This is not a trivial matter for the patients who may be subjected to such procedures. However, as Greene and Obrez[101] have observed, there is no medical justification for repositioning the mandible in most dentate people. Having a symptomatic TMD problem does not change that fact, unless the clinician buys into a concept of occlusal causes for such problems. However, as stated many times in this article and elsewhere, the evidence at this time does not support this outdated concept. Almost all current authoritative guidelines for treating TMDs have stated that conservative treatment is the appropriate strategy for most patients,[102,103] including the proper use of OAs in treating them. As previously described in the sections on treating both TMJ and muscular problems, there are many reasonable applications for OAs and all of them are based on conservative concepts of therapy. At this time, clinicians should be moving beyond the old concepts of appliance therapy and related occlusal modifications so that current and future TMD patients can receive

the potential benefits of wearing an OA without the risk of having unnecessary irreversible procedures done on them.

ACKNOWLEDGMENTS

The authors would like to thank Dr Karen Raphael for her helpful discussions about several issues in this article.

REFERENCES

1. Gelb ML, Gelb H. Mandibular orthopedic repositioning therapy. Cranio Clin Int 1991;1:81–98.
2. Shankland WE. Nociceptive trigeminal inhibition—tension suppression system: a method of preventing migraine and tension headaches. Compend Contin Educ Dent 2002;23:105–8.
3. Al Quran FA, Kamal MS. Anterior midline point stop device (AMPS) in the treatment of myogenous TMDs: comparison with the stabilization splint and control group. Oral Surg Oral Med Oral Pathol Oral Radiol Endod 2006;101:741–7.
4. Baad-Hansen L, Jadidi F, Castrillon E, et al. Effect of a nociceptive trigeminal inhibitory splint on electromyographic activity in jaw closing muscles during sleep. J Oral Rehabil 2007;34:105–11.
5. Hylander WL. An experimental analysis of temporomandibular joint reaction force in Macaques. Am J Phys Anthropol 1979;51:433–56.
6. Brehnan K, Boyd RL, Laskin J, et al. Direct measurement of loads at the temporomandibular joint. J Dent Res 1981;60:1820–4.
7. Nitzan DW. Intraarticular pressure in the functioning human temporomandibular joint and its alteration by uniform elevation of the occlusal plane. J Oral Maxillofac Surg 1994;52:671–9 [discussion: 679–80].
8. Casares G, Thomas A, Carmona J, et al. The influence of oral stabilization appliances in intraarticular pressure of the temporomandibular joint. Cranio 2014;32:219–23.
9. Smith DM, McLachlan KR, McCall WD Jr. A numerical model of temporomandibular joint loading. J Dent Res 1986;65:1046–52.
10. Toro-Ibacache V, O'Higgins P. The effect of varying jaw-elevator muscle forces on a finite element model of a human cranium. Anat Rec (Hoboken) 2016;299:828–39.
11. Korioth TWP, Hannam AG. Effect of bilateral asymmetric tooth clenching on load distribution at the mandibular condyles. J Prosthet Dent 1990;64:69–73.
12. Rues S, Lenz J, Turp J, et al. Muscle and joint forces under variable equilibrium states of the mandible. Clin Oral Investig 2011;15:737–47.

13. Perez del Palomar A, Santana-Penin U, Mora-Bermúdez MJ, et al. Clenching TMJs-loads increases in partial edentates: a 3-D finite element study. Ann Biomed Eng 2008;36:1014–23.

14. Ettlin DA, Mang H, Colombo V, et al. Stereometric assessment of TMJ space variation by occlusal splints. J Dent Res 2008;87:877–81.

15. Ito T, Gibbs CH, Marguelles-Bonnet R, et al. Loading on the temporomandibular joints with five occlusal conditions. J Prosthet Dent 1986;56:478–84.

16. Hattori Y, Satoh C, Seki S, et al. Occlusal and TMJ loads in subjects with experimentally shortened dental arches. J Dent Res 2003;82:532–6.

17. Breul R, Mall G, Landgraf J, et al. Biomechanical analysis of stress distribution in the human temporomandibular-joint. Ann Anat 1999;181:55–60.

18. Beek M, Aarnts MP, Koolstra JH, et al. Dynamic properties of the human temporomandibular joint disc. J Dent Res 2001;80:876–80.

19. Dawson PE. Evaluation, diagnosis, and treatment of occlusal problems. 2nd edition. St Louis (MO): Mosby; 1989. p. 28–55, 434–41.

20. Dawson PE. Functional occlusion from TMJ to smile design. 2nd edition. St Louis (MO): Mosby; 2007. p. 36–7.

21. Beek M, Koolstra JH, van Ruijven LJ, et al. Three-dimensional finite element analysis of the cartilaginous structures in the human temporomandibular joint. J Dent Res 2001;80:1913–8.

22. Kubein-Meesenburg D, Fanghanel J, Ihlow D, et al. Functional state of the mandible and rolling-gliding characteristics in the TMJ. Ann Anat 2007;189:393–6.

23. Stankovic S, Vlajkovic S, Boskovic M, et al. Morphological and biomechanical features of the temporomandibular disc: an overview of recent findings. Arch Oral Biol 2013;58:1475–82.

24. Milam SB, Schmitz JP. Molecular biology of temporomandibular joint disorders. J Oral Maxillofac Surg 1995;53:1448–54.

25. Milam SB, Zardentata G, Schmitz JB. Oxidative stress and degenerative temporomandibular joint disease: a proposed hypothesis. J Oral Maxillfac Surg 1998;56:214–23.

26. Hylander WL. The human mandible: lever or link? Am J Phys Anthropol 1975;43:227–42.

27. Kurita K, Westesson PL, Yuasa H, et al. Natural course of untreated symptomatic temporomandibular joint disc displacement without reduction. J Dent Res 1998;77:361–5.

28. Breul R. Biomechanical analysis of stress distribution in the temporomandibular joint. Ann Anat 2007;189:329–35.

29. Koc D, Dogan A, Bek B. Bite force and influential factors on bite force measurements: a literature review. Eur J Dent 2010;4:223–32.

30. Moncayo S. Biomechanics of pivoting appliances. J Orofac Pain 1994;8:190–6.

31. Demling A, Fauska K, Ismail F, et al. A comparison of change in condylar position in asymptomatic volunteers utilizing a stabilization and a pivot appliance. Cranio 2009;27:54–61.

32. Behr M, Stebner K, Kolbeck C, et al. Outcomes of temporomandibular joint disorder therapy: observations over 13 years. Acta Odontol Scand 2007;65:249–53.

33. Okeson JP. The effects of hard and soft occlusal splints on nocturnal bruxism. J Am Dent Assoc 1987;114:788–91.

34. Cruz-Reyes RA, Martinez-Aragon I, Guerro-Arias RE, et al. Influence of occlusal stabilization splints and soft occlusal splints on the electromyographic pattern, in basal state and at the end of six weeks treatment in patients with bruxism. Acta Odontol Latinoam 2011;24:66–74.

35. Serra CM, Manns AE. Bite force measurements with hard and soft bite surfaces. J Oral Rehabil 2013;40:563–8.

36. Faulkner JA. Terminology for contractions of muscles during shortening, while isometric, and during lengthening. J Appl Physiol (1985) 2003;95:455–9.

37. Williamson EH, Lundquist DO. Anterior guidance: its effect on electromyographic activity of the temporal and masseter muscles. J Prosthet Dent 1983;49:816–23.

38. Conti PC, dos Santos CN, Kogawa EM, et al. The treatment of painful temporomandibular joint clicking with oral splints: a randomized clinical trial. J Am Dent Assoc 2006;137:1108–14.

39. Staplemann H, Turp J. The NTI-tss device for the therapy of bruxism, temporomandibular disorders, and headache – where do we stand? A qualitative systematic review of the literature. BMC Oral Health 2008;8:22.

40. Santana-Mora U, Martinez-Insua A, Santana-Penin U, et al. Muscular activity during isometric incisal biting. J Biomech 2014;47:3891–7.

41. Huang GJ, LeResche L, Critchlow CW, et al. Risk factors for diagnostic subgroups of painful temporomandibular disorders (TMD). J Dent Res 2002;81:284–8.

42. Commisso MS, Martinez-Reina J, Mayo J. A study of the temporomandibular joint during bruxism. Int J Oral Sci 2014;6:116–23.

43. Okano N, Baba K, Ohyama T. The influence of altered occlusal guidance on condylar displacement during submaximal clenching. J Oral Rehabil 2005;32:714–9.

44. Türp JC, Komine F, Hugger A. Efficacy of stabilization splints for the management of patients with masticatory muscle pain: a qualitative systematic review. Clin Oral Investig 2004;8:179–95.

45. Dao TT, Lavigne GJ. Oral splints: the crutches for temporomandibular disorders and bruxism? Crit Rev Oral Biol Med 1998;9:345–61.

46. Ziad AA, Gray RJ, Davies SJ, et al. Stabilization splint therapy for the treatment of temporomandibular myofascial pain: a systematic review. J Dent Educ 2005;69:1242–50.

47. Raphael K, Sirois D, Janal MN, et al. Sleep bruxism and myofascial temporomandibular disorders: a laboratory-based polysomnographic investigation. J Am Dent Assoc 2012;143:1223–31.

48. Schiffman E, Ohrbach R, Truelove E, et al. Diagnostic Criteria for Temporomandibular Disorders (DC/TMD) for Clinical and Research Applications: recommendations of the International RDC/TMD Consortium Network and Orofacial Pain Special Interest Group. J Oral Facial Pain Headache 2014; 28:6–27.

49. Limchaichana N, Nillson H, Ekberg EC, et al. Clinical diagnoses and MRI findings in patients with TMD pain. J Oral Rehabil 2007;34:237–45.

50. Hebert-Blouin MN, Tubbs S, Carmichael S, et al. Hilton's law revisited. Clin Anat 2014;27:548–55.

51. Landulpho AB, Silva WAB, Silva FA, et al. Electromyographic evaluation of masseter and anterior temporalis muscles in patients with temporomandibular disorders following interocclusal appliance treatment. J Oral Rehabil 2004;31:95–8.

52. Ekberg EC, Vallon D, Nilner M. Occlusal appliance therapy in patients with temporomandibular disorders: a double-blind controlled study in a short term perspective. Acta Odontol Scand 1998;56:122–8.

53. De Leeuw JRJ, Steenks WJG, Ros AM, et al. Assessment of treatment outcome in patients with craniomandibular dysfunction. J Oral Rehabil 1994;21:655–66.

54. Wilkes CH. Internal derangements of the temporomandibular joint. Pathological variations. Northwest Dent 1990;69:25–32.

55. Aidar L, Abrahão M, Yamashita H, et al. Herbst appliance therapy and temporomandibular joint disc position: a prospective longitudinal magnetic resonance imaging study. Am J Orthod Dentofacial Orthop 2006;129:486–96.

56. Pliska BT, Hyejin N, Chen H, et al. Obstructive sleep apnea and mandibular advancement splints: occlusal effects and progression of changes associated with a decade of treatment. J Clin Sleep Med 2014;10:1285–91.

57. Perez C, de Leeuw R, Okeson JP, et al. The incidence and prevalence of temporomandibular disorders and posterior open bite in patients receiving mandibular advancement device therapy for obstructive sleep apnea. Sleep Breath 2013;17: 323–32.

58. Elving L, Helkimo M, Magnusson T. Prevalence of different temporomandibular joint sounds, with emphasis on disc-displacement, in patients with temporomandibular disorders and controls. Swed Dent J 2002;26:9–19.

59. Keeling S, McGorray S, Wheeler T, et al. Risk factors associated with temporomandibular joint sounds in children 6 to 12 years of age. Am J Orthod Dentofacial Orthop 1994;105:279–87.

60. Magnusson T, Egermark I, Carlsson GE. A longitudinal epidemiological study of signs and symptoms of temporomandibular disorders from 15 to 35 years of age. J Orofac Pain 2000;14: 310–9.

61. Westesson PL, Paesani D. MR imaging of the TMJ: decreased signal from the retrodiscal tissue. Oral Surg Oral Med Oral Pathol 1993;76:631–5.

62. Suenaga S, Sonoda S, Oku T, et al. MRI of the temporomandibular joint disk and posterior disk attachment before and after nonsurgical treatment. J Comput Assist Tomogr 1997;21:892–6.

63. Hall HD. Intra-articular disk displacement part II: its significant role in temporomandibular joint pathology. J Oral Maxillofac Surg 1995;53:1073–9.

64. Nickerson JW, Moystad A. Observations on individuals with bilateral condylar remodeling. J Craniomandibular Pract 1982;1:21–7.

65. Hall HD, Nickerson JW. Is it time to pay more attention to disc position? J Orofac Pain 1994;8:90–6.

66. Vincent KR, Conrad BP, Fregly BJ, et al. The pathophysiology of osteoarthritis: a mechanical perspective on the knee joint. PM R 2012;4(5 Suppl):S3–9.

67. Gavish A, Halachimi M, Winocur E, et al. Oral habits and their association with signs and symptoms of temporomandibular disorders in adolescent girls. J Oral Rehabil 2000;27:22–32.

68. Farrar WB. Diagnosis and treatment of anterior dislocation of the articular disc. N Y J Dent 1971; 41:348–51.

69. Summer JD, Westesson PL. Mandibular repositioning can be effective in treatment of reducing TMJ disk displacement. A long-term clinical and MR imaging follow-up. Cranio 1997;15:107–20.

70. Simmons HC. Guidelines for anterior repositioning appliance therapy for the management of craniofacial pain and TMD. Cranio 2005;23:300–5.

71. Okeson JP. Long-term treatment of disk-interference disorders of the temporomandibular joint with anterior repositioning occlusal splints. J Prosthet Dent 1988;60:611–6.

72. Zamburlini I, Austin D. Long-term results of appliance therapies in anterior disk displacement with reduction: a review of the literature. Cranio 1991; 9(4):361–8.

73. Eberhard D, Bantleon HP, Steger W. The efficacy of anterior repositioning splint therapy studied by magnetic resonance imaging. Eur J Orthod 2002; 24:343–52.

74. Conti PC, Corrêa AS, Lauris JR, et al. Management of painful temporomandibular joint clicking with different intraoral devices and counseling: a controlled study. J Appl Oral Sci 2015;23:529–35.

75. Chen HM, Liu MC, Yap AU-J, et al. Physiological effects of anterior repositioning splint on temporomandibular joint disc displacement: a quantitative analysis. J Oral Rehabil 2017;44:664–72.

76. Tecco S, Festa F, Salini V, et al. Treatment of joint pain and joint noises associated with a recent TMJ internal derangement: a comparison of an anterior repositioning splint, a full-arch maxillary stabilization splint, and an untreated control group. Cranio 2004;22:209–19.

77. Chang SW, Ching-Ya C, Jau Rong L, et al. Treatment effects of maxillary flat occlusal splints for painful clicking of the temporomandibular joint. Kaohsiung J Med Sci 2010;26:299–307.

78. Lee SH, Yoon HJ. MRI Findings of patients with temporomandibular joint internal derangement: before and after performance of arthrocentesis and stabilization splint. J Oral Maxillofac Surg 2009;67:314–7.

79. Barkin S, Weinberg S. Internal derangements of the temporomandibular joint: the role of arthroscopic surgery and arthrocentesis. J Can Dent Assoc 2000;66:199–203.

80. Conti AC, Pegoraro LF, Araujo CR. Partial time use of anterior repositioning splints in the management of TMJ pain and dysfunction: a one year controlled study. J Appl Oral Sci 2005;13:345–50.

81. Dao TTT, Lavigne GJ, Charbonneau A, et al. The efficacy of oral splints in the treatment of myofascial pain of the jaw muscles: a controlled clinical trial. Pain 1994;56:85–94.

82. Gavish A, Winocur E, Ventura YS, et al. Effect of stabilization splint therapy on pain during chewing in patients suffering from myofascial pain. J Oral Rehabil 2002;29:1181–6.

83. Ekberg EC, Vallon D, Nilner M. The efficacy of appliance therapy in patients with temporomandibular disorders of mainly myogenous origin. A randomized, controlled, short-term study. J Orofac Pain 2003;17:133–9.

84. Forssell H, Kalso E, Koskela P. Occlusal treatments in temporomandibular disorders: a qualitative systematic review of randomized controlled trials. Pain 1999;83:549–60.

85. Kreiner M, Betancor E, Clark GT. Occlusal stabilization appliances. Evidence of their efficacy. J Am Dent Assoc 2001;132:770–7.

86. Delsnyder J, Colina T, Elsemary N, et al. Stabilization appliances as treatment for myogenous temporomandibular disorders: a systematic review and meta-analysis. Open J Dent Oral Med 2017;5:72–84.

87. Klasser GD, Greene CS. Oral appliances in the management of temporomandibular disorders. Oral Surg Oral Med Oral Pathol Oral Radiol Endod 2009;107:212–23.

88. Raphael KG, Marbach JJ. Widespread pain and the effectiveness of oral splints in myofascial face pain. J Am Dent Assoc 2001;132:305–16.

89. Lund JP, Donga R, Widmer CG, et al. The pain-adaptation model: a discussion of the relationship between chronic musculoskeletal pain and motor activity. Can J Physiol Pharmacol 1991;69:683–94.

90. Murray GM, Peck CC. Orofacial pain and jaw muscle activity: a new model. J Orofac Pain 2007;21: 263–78.

91. Okeson JP. Occlusal appliance therapy. In: Okeson JP, editor. Management of temporomandibular disorders and occlusion. St Louis (MO): Mosby; 2008. p. 492–4.

92. Ramfjord SP. Bruxism, a clinical and electromyographic study. J Am Dent Assoc 1961;62:21–44.

93. Shore NA. Occlusal equilibration and temporomandibular joint dysfunction. Philadelphia: Lippincott; 1959.

94. Karl PJ, Foley TF. Use of a deprogramming appliance to obtain centric relation. Angle Orthod 1999;69:117–24.

95. McKee J. Comparing condylar positions achieved through bimanual manipulation to condylar positions achieved through masticatory muscle contraction against an anterior deprogrammer: a pilot study. J Prosthet Dent 2005;94:389–93.

96. Jayne D. A deprogrammer for occlusal analysis and simplified case mounting. J Cosmetic Dent 2006;21(4):96–102.

97. Jankelson B. Neuromuscular aspects of occlusion. Dent Clin North Am 1979;23:157–68.

98. Cooper BC. The role of bioelectric instrumentation in the documentation and management of temporomandibular disorders. Oral Surg Oral Med Oral Pathol Oral Radiol Endod 1997;83:91–100.

99. Tripodakis AP, Smulow JB, Mehta NR, et al. Clinical study of location and reproducibility of three mandibular positions in relation to body posture and muscle function. J Prosthet Dent 1995;73: 190–8.

100. Rinchuse DJ, Kandasamy S. Centric relation: an historical and contemporary orthodontic perspective. J Am Dent Assoc 2006;137:494–501.

101. Greene CS, Obrez A. Treating temporomandibular disorders with permanent mandibular repositioning: is it medically necessary? Oral Surg Oral Med Oral Pathol Oral Radiol 2015;119:489–98.

102. American Association for Dental Research. Temporomandibular disorders (TMD). Adopted 2010. Available at: www.aadronline.org/i4a/pages/index. cfm?pageid=3465. Accessed December 12, 2017.

103. Greene CS. Managing the care of patients with temporomandibular disorders: a new guideline for care. J Am Dent Assoc 2010;141:1086–8.

The Efficacy of Pharmacologic Treatment of Temporomandibular Disorders

Gary M. Heir, DMD

KEYWORDS

- Pharmacotherapy • Temporomandibular disorders • Nociception • Peripheral sensitization
- Myofascial pain

KEY POINTS

- Successful pharmacologic management of temporomandibular disorders depends on an understanding of the pain mechanisms involved.
- Knowing why to prescribe is as important as knowing what to prescribe.
- The source of the pain determines the therapeutic choice.
- Improper diagnosis is a common cause of therapeutic failure.
- A common mistake is the use of peripherally acting analgesics for centrally mediated pain.

INTRODUCTION

Epidemiologic data indicates that 33% of the general population has at least one symptom of a temporomandibular disorder (TMD); 6% to 7% have TMDs severe enough to seek treatment. Pharmacologic therapy is commonly used as part of the management of these conditions. To accomplish this successfully requires an understanding of the pain mechanisms involved. Failure to understand these mechanisms leads to inaccurate diagnoses and ineffective, delayed, or harmful treatment.

Although it is the responsibility of the provider to accurately diagnose and treat the various TMDs, it is equally important to know when not to treat. Knowing why a treatment is provided is as important as knowing how it should be administered. Equally important is knowing what the medication does to the patient and what the patient does to the medication. This includes knowing the therapeutic target of any medication prescribed, its side effects, any drug interactions, and the medical history of the patient.

This article provides a brief review of pain mechanisms, identifies pharmacologic targets, and discusses the efficacy of pharmacotherapy routinely used for pain associated with TMDs and orofacial pain disorders.

NOCICEPTION

Nociceptors in the temporomandibular joint (TMJ) and masticatory muscles, when activated, transduce the stimulus into an electrical signal that is transmitted via an action potential to the trigeminal nuclei. As nociceptors synapse within the dorsal horn, they pass the signal on to second-order neurons via neurotransmitters released into the synaptic space. Activation of second-order neurons transmits noxious impulses to various sites within the central nervous system and brain, primarily through the medial and lateral thalamus, where

Disclosure: The author has nothing to disclose.
Department of Diagnostic Sciences, Center for Temporomandiublar Disorders and Orofacial Pain, Rutgers School of Dental Medicine, Room D880, 110 Bergen Street, Newark, NJ 07101, USA
E-mail address: heirgm@sdm.rutgers.edu

Oral Maxillofacial Surg Clin N Am 30 (2018) 279–285
https://doi.org/10.1016/j.coms.2018.05.001

they are then distributed for further processing. Medications that interrupt or reduce the release of neurotransmitters at the synapse between the first- and second-order neurons inhibit or modulate the pain and thus provide a target for its control.

The brain constructs a scenario from the information received via the nociceptors and determines if the stimulus is harmful, the degree of pain, and the action necessary to minimize the threat of potential injury. Contributions of memory of similar events, or emotional overlay, can result in a diminished ability to inhibit noxious input and pain facilitation by affecting the descending pain modulating system. This system regulates the release of excitatory and faciliatory neuropeptides, endogenous opioids, and has other functions that influence the perception of pain.

This simplistic description points to several targets for medications, such as peripheral receptors, primary afferent neurons, pain inhibition at the dorsal horn, the descending pain inhibitory system, and the brain.

PERIPHERAL AND CENTRAL SENSITIZATION

In a patient with a TMJ or myofascial pain there is a release of inflammatory mediators that sensitize the peripheral nociceptors. In this case, the administration of nonsteroidal anti-inflammatory drugs (NSAIDs), acting peripherally, reduces inflammation, decreases primary afferent sensitization, and results in pain reduction.

The process of peripheral sensitization typically ends when the source of pain is withdrawn, or the healing process is complete. However, in some cases, pain persists. In such instances, chronic noxious signals reach the central nervous system resulting in a phenomenon referred to as central sensitization, a process of strengthening synaptic connections and signal transmissions. Central sensitization results in a cascade of events, such as amplification of noxious signals, while at the same time reducing the efficiency of pain inhibition. This scenario points to additional pharmacologic targets. Treatment with anti-inflammatory drugs alone results in only partial success because the additional targets are more centrally located. The original injury may even have resolved, but central sensitization continues to drive chronic pain. Therefore, knowing the target of the treatment and classifying analgesics by the site of action, results in a better outcome (**Box 1**).

CHRONIC PAIN

If pain assumes a chronic nature, more centrally mediated mechanisms take effect, for which

---

Box 1
Classification of analgesics by site of action

- Inhibits peripheral sensitization
  - NSAIDs
    - Cyclooxygenase 1 and 2 inhibitors
      - Blocks prostaglandin synthesis
      - Blocks or reduces afferent nerve transmission
  - Anticonvulsants
    - Gabanoids (neurontin, pregabalin)
      - Controls calcium influx
      - Reduces release of sympathetic excitatory amino acids
  - Antiepileptic drugs
    - Carbamazepine
      - Axonal membrane stabilizer
      - Sodium channel blocker
      - May stimulate release of serotonin and possibly act as a reuptake inhibitor facilitating pain inhibition
- Facilitates endogenous inhibitory mechanisms
  - Antidepressants
    - Serotonin reuptake inhibitors
    - Serotonin/noradrenaline reuptake inhibitors
  - Reduces signal transmission at the dorsal horn
- Presynaptic or post-synaptic inhibitory effect
  - Opioids

---

peripherally acting analgesics have less efficacy. The clinician must recognize the involved alterations in pain characteristics, such as quality, duration, and intensity, as peripheral pain becomes more continuous, diffuse, and difficult to localize. In such instances, the possibility of new targets for treatment emerges.

Chronic pain is not a symptom. It is a disease, often amplified by a sense of unpredictability of treatment. The lack of an understanding of the meaning of the symptoms, and negative expectations of recovery, lead to anxiety and depression, embellishing the pain response. Pain is perceived at the original site even though healing may be complete and no additional pathology has occurred. Stimuli are amplified, causing the perception of nonnoxious input as painful in this scenario, and peripherally acting analgesic/anti-inflammatory drugs serve little purpose.

MODULATION AND THE PAIN INHIBITORY SYSTEMS

Through a series of complex interactions within the brain, cognition of a noxious stimulus is analyzed against memories, assessed for emotional context, and finally processed. Once the information is processed, the output may be emotional, sensory, or both. Physiologic changes also take place that can influence the perception of pain depending on the context in which the pathology occurs.[1,2]

Downregulating pain inhibitory pathways in the trigeminal nucleus caudalis affects the transmission of signals from the primary to the secondary neurons. Significant contributors to this process of pain inhibition include noradrenaline, serotonin, γ-aminobutyric acid, and endogenous opioids. Targeting these neuromodulators is a strategy for controlling peripheral pain.

PHARMACOLOGIC TREATMENT OF TEMPOROMANDIBULAR DISORDER PAIN
Nonsteroidal Anti-inflammatory Drugs

Achieving pain relief for an arthrogenous or myogenous TMD is achieved with the use of peripherally acting NSAIDs, such as salicylates, acetaminophen, and ibuprofen. They offer three basic effects: (1) analgesic; (2) anti-inflammatory; and (3) with the exception of acetaminophen, antipyretic.[3] These medications act on cyclooxygenase (COX)-1 and 2. Acting peripherally, NSAIDs block prostaglandin synthesis resulting in reduced sensitization and excitation of peripheral nociceptors.[4]

Another function of NSAIDs is reduction of secondary hyperalgesia caused by reduction of facilitated pain states produced by peripheral injury and inflammation and by direct activation of spinal glutamate and substance P receptors.[5] Guidelines for the use of NSAIDs are listed in **Box 2**.

Acetaminophen

Acetaminophen is perhaps the most commonly used NSAID. It acts on COX-2 and COX-3. It also blocks prostaglandin formation in the central nervous system, acts on the endocannabinoid system, and influences central nervous system serotonin.[6,7]

Acetaminophen is safe for use in elderly patients, where it is the drug of choice. It also may be used in the presence of asthma, gastric irritation, and at regular strength (2–2.5 g/d) in the presence of liver or kidney disease (**Table 1**). However,

---

Box 2
Traditional NSAID and COXIB treatment guidelines

- Prescribe the lowest effective dose for the shortest period of time
- Chronic pain: consider as required dosing only and review regularly
- Advise patient regarding potential toxicities
- Arrange appropriate monitoring: renal function, blood pressure, liver function
- Patients on aspirin: avoid NSAIDs and COXIBs where possible
- Renal insufficiency: avoid where possible and in those with glomerular filtration rate less than 30 mL/min
- Hepatic insufficiency: avoid where possible and diclofenac in particular
- Anticoagulation: avoid NSAIDs in patients on warfarin or heparin

Adapted from Mehta P, Mason JC. NSAIDs and COXIBs: the stomach, the heart and the brain: Reports on the Rheumatic Diseases. Spring 2010;6(5). Available at: http://www.arthritisresearchuk.org/health-professionals-and-students/reports/topical-reviews/topical-reviews-spring-2010.aspx; with permission.

---

acetaminophen is hepatotoxic. For this reason, the Food and Drug Administration limits all acetaminophen-containing over-the-counter medications to 325 mg per dose. The recommended daily dose for healthy individuals should not exceed 3000 mg. Severe liver damage can occur if more than 3000 mg is taken in a 24-hour period. Its use may be contraindicated in individuals with liver disease and alcoholics. Overuse of acetaminophen is common because of the number of preparations that include this medication. For example, cold and flu medications, allergy preparations, and muscle pain relievers may contain acetaminophen. The patient may not readily share the use of these over-the-counter remedies during the history-taking, because often they do not consider them medications if purchased outside the realm of a pharmacy.

COXIBs

COXIBs represent another category of NSAIDs/COX inhibitors that affect a third COX isozyme, COX-3. It is found in the cerebral cortex and is selectively inhibited by the analgesic and antipyretic effects of medications, such as acetaminophen, and other NSAIDs.[5] This may explain the efficacy of acetaminophen in decreasing pain.

Table 1
Acetaminophen overview

Drug	Indications	Possible Side Effects	Potential Interactions	Precautions and Contraindications
Acetaminophen	• Pain • Fever	• ↑ Bilirubin • ↑ Alkaline phosphatase • Skin reactions • Liver toxicity • Hypertension	• Barbiturates • Carbamazepine • Cholestyramine • Isoniazid • Warfarin	Precautions • G6PD deficiency • Chronic alcoholics • Hepatic/renal impairment Contraindications • Hypersensitivity • Severe liver impairment/disease

Abbreviation: G6PD, glucose-6-phosphate dehydrogenase.
Adapted from Food and Drug Administration Nonprescription Drugs Advisory Committee, September 19, 2002. Available at: http://wayback.archive-it.org/7993/20170403222314/https://www.fda.gov/ohrms/dockets/ac/cder02.htm#Nonprescription Drugs. Accessed June 7, 2018.

There have been reports of cardiovascular risk leading to the withdrawal of some COXIBs from the marketplace. The guidelines for the use of COXIBs are listed in **Box 2**.

TREATING TEMPOROMANDIBULAR DISORDER PAIN WITHOUT OPIOIDS

A review article in the *Journal of the American Dental Association*[8] addressing the treatment of dental pain following third molar extraction noted that 325 mg of acetaminophen taken with 200 mg of ibuprofen provides better pain relief than oral opioids. It concluded, "The results of the quantitative systematic reviews indicated that the ibuprofen-acetaminophen combination may be a more effective analgesic, with fewer untoward effects than many of the currently available opioid-containing formulations commonly prescribed for pain in the dental setting." This includes treatment of acute TMDs.

TREATMENT OF CHRONIC NEUROPATHIC PAIN

Neuropathic pain is not a diagnosis, but describes a clinical condition.[9] It can result from injury to peripheral efferent nerves, loss of descending inhibitory effects, diminished pain inhibition or increased facilitation at the level of the brainstem, or a heightened awareness of pain at higher levels in the cortex. Anti-inflammatory drugs and analgesics have little effect. Opioids are efficacious, but only at higher doses. The treatment of neuropathic pain requires recognition of additional targets and is based on the proposed mechanism of the pain. Possible mechanisms and classification of medications are listed in **Box 3**.

Direct trauma to a nerve can result in an upregulation of sodium channels at the site of trauma. Ectopic discharge can occur, with action potentials reporting noxious impulses to the central nervous system. Tricyclic antidepressants can stabilize sodium channels, reducing ectopic activity.[10]

Neuronal injury can also result in the upregulation of cholinergic receptors. Following trauma, α_1 and α_2 adrenergic receptors are expressed on sensory neurons and postganglionic sympathetic terminals. Studies indicate that a chronic form of neuropathic pain increased by activity of the sympathetic nervous system, sympathetically maintained pain, is mediated by α_1 and α_2 adrenergic receptors. Increased sympathetic activity raises the levels of circulating norepinephrine, activating these cholinergic receptors and resulting in the propagation of noxious impulses from the affected afferent neurons.[11–13] The analgesic effect of tricyclic antidepressants occurs by blocking α_1 and α_2 receptors.[14]

Patients with chronic pain develop inefficiency of the pain inhibitory system.[15] A primary neuromodulator is serotonin. Serotonin is released from the descending pathways at the dorsal horn and is immediately taken back into the cell from which it was released (serotonin reuptake). This process is regulated by the descending pain modulating system, which becomes inefficient in chronic pain conditions. Tricyclic antidepressants, referred to as serotonin reuptake inhibitors, make serotonin more available by inhibiting its reuptake after release into the synapse. By remaining in the synapse for a longer period it makes pain inhibition more efficient. Selective serotonin reuptake inhibitors have a similar effect but are less effective pain inhibitors. They can induce nocturnal bruxism in some patients if taken close to retiring for sleep.[16]

Box 3
Mechanisms of neuropathic pain and suppressive medications

- Abnormal Na+ channel expression
  - Occurs in the presence of direct trauma to a nerve or nerves
    - Spontaneous or ectopic action potentials emanating from the site of injury may occur
    - The following classes of medications act as cell membrane stabilizers and reduce the active of sodium channels
      - Tricyclic antidepressants
      - Serotonin-noradrenaline reuptake inhibitors
      - Local and topical anesthetics
      - Some antiepileptic drugs
- Increased glutamate receptor activity
  - Takes place in the dorsal horn at the connection between the primary afferent and second-order neuron; synaptic strength is increased
    - N-Methyl-D-aspartate antagonists
    - α-Amino-3-hydroxy-5-methyl-4-isoxazolepropionic acid receptor antagonist
- Altered gabapentin inhibition
  - Pain inhibition is affected
    - Gabapentinergic agents
    - Anticonvulsants
    - Baclofen
- Calcium influx
  - Excessive release of neurotransmitters is diminished
    - Gabapentin
    - Pregablin

INTRA-ARTICULAR INJECTIONS

Intra-articular injections into the TMJ to control pain and inflammation have been used in two ways: alone or combined with arthrocentesis. The most commonly used agents have been the corticosteroids (betamethasone, methylprednisolone, triamcinolone, dexamethasone) and sodium hyaluronate. When used following arthrocentesis for treating an internal derangement, most studies have shown no better results with either agent than with only arthrocentesis. This may be caused by arthrocentesis alone being able to resolve the problem.

When injection of a corticosteroid alone into the TMJ for managing the acute symptoms of osteoarthritis was compared with the use of sodium hyaluronate, the results showed them to be equally effective. However, it has been reported that the antianabolic effect of steroids can result in frequently repeated injections actually producing further degenerative changes in the joint. On this basis, it is recommended that intra-articular steroids not be used more frequently than every 3 to 4 months. Accidental intracutaneous or subcutaneous injection can also cause local skin atrophy. Although sodium hyaluronate is more expensive than the corticosteroids, repeated injections have not been associated with similar condylar changes.

Intra-articular injection of morphine or platelet-rich plasma into the arthritic TMJ has also been reported, but there are insufficient studies available at this time to confirm their effectiveness.

MUSCLE PAIN AND ITS PHARMACOTHERAPY

There is a misconception that muscle relaxants act directly on muscle tissue resulting in some specific effect. This is not the case; they act more systemically than on specific muscle targets.

Terms used to describe muscle dysfunction include spasticity and spasm. Muscle spasticity is characterized by rigidity (hypertonia), exaggerated tendon jerks (hyperreflexia), and paralysis. Specifically, as seen in cerebral palsy, multiple sclerosis, and stroke, the patient may suffer from a disabling inability to straighten joints.

Spasms are not necessarily caused by systemic disorders but can be caused by local factors involving affected muscle groups. Spasms are more common than spasticity, and may be associated with headache, back or neck pain, or other conditions caused by chronic pain emanating from muscle tissues. In the case of spasm, the muscles are not excessively tense, nor do they demonstrate hyperreflexia.

Myofascial pain (MFP) is deep, dull, and constant, with a sense of tightness or pressure. It is increased by functional activity of the involved structures. The presence of myofascial trigger points confirms the diagnosis of MFP. It is estimated that 85% of patients presenting to chronic pain centers suffer from MFP caused by trigger points (TrPs) as the primary diagnosis.[17] The underlying pathology is unclear, but MFP is associated with local muscle injury or abuse, trauma, overuse, and abnormal posture to name a few comorbidities. Local contracture develops, and a few motor end plates become dysfunctional. Miniature motor end plate potentials occur secondary to acetylcholine leakage from motor neurons and local contracture forming TrPs follows.[18] A second hypothesis suggests that the formation of TrPs is the result of a central nervous system component. The intensified pain state in chronic myofascial pain patients may be associated with abnormal neural activity suggesting central sensitization, and the possibility of a neurotransmitter disruption between the motor nerve and target muscle.[19]

Fibromyalgia syndrome is often confused with MFP. Fibromyalgia syndrome represents a dysregulation of the pain modulation system. Pain of fibromyalgia syndrome may resemble MFP, and there is speculation that myofascial pain may be a centrally mediated sensitization disorder. Therefore, although they may seem similar clinically, they may not respond the same to therapy.

A commonly used local therapeutic agent for muscle pain is cyclobenzaprine, which is structurally similar to the tricyclic antidepressants. Although not an antidepressant, it has a sedative effect, causing a sense of relaxation. It is contraindicated in patients on monoamine oxidase inhibitors and, because of its atropine-like action, used with caution in patients with a history of urinary retention, angle-closure glaucoma, and increased intraocular pressure.

Most of the commonly used muscle relaxants used for MFP have similar actions to cyclobenzaprine. These include the following:

- Acting primarily in the brain to relax skeletal muscle by unknown mechanisms
- All have a general depressant effect on the central nervous system
- They may reduce polysynaptic reflex activity in the spinal cord
- They decrease alpha motor neuron excitability

Muscle relaxants are grouped into four categories by the mechanism of action[20]:

- Neuromuscular-blocking drugs
  ○ Reduce muscle contractility
- Antispasticity drugs
  ○ Reduce muscle cramping and tightness in neurologic disorders and spinal cord injury and disease
- Antispasm drugs
  ○ Prevent use-related minor muscle spasms
- Motor nerve blocker (botulinum toxin)
  ○ Blepharospasm and strabismus
  ○ Elective cosmetic purposes

Examples include the following:

Diazepam
- Acts on Cl^- channels, enhances GABA-A receptors, and causes inhibition at presynaptic and postsynaptic sites in the spinal cord
- Acts in the brain as a hypnotic and sedative

Baclofen
- Acts on K^+ channels
- Presynaptically at GABA-B receptors in the spinal cord to reduce transmitter, releases K^+
- Antispasmodic

Tizanidine
- Acts presynaptically at α_2 adrenergic receptors
- Inhibits spinal motor neurons

Dantrolene
- Reduces Ca^{++} release from sacroplasmic reticulum/pathologic contraction

Botulinum toxin
- Prevents ACh release

There is no clear consensus on the efficacy of botulinum toxin (Botox) for treatment of chronic MFP (see Daniel M. Laskin's article, "The Use of Botulinum Toxin for the Treatment of Myofascial Pain in the Masticatory Muscles," in this issue). Randomized controlled studies have shown that botulinum toxin is no more effective than dry needling or other solutions. A Cochrane systematic review of nine trials (503 participants) found that botulinum toxin was no better than the placebo (saline) for patients with subacute or chronic neck pain. Available evidence did not support the use of botulinum toxin either as a monotherapy or in combination with any other treatment in patients with subacute or chronic neck pain.[21,22]

CAUSES OF PHARMACOLOGIC TREATMENT FAILURE

If a patient does not respond to treatment within a reasonable time, the clinician must question the accuracy of the diagnosis or the efficacy of the treatment. The diagnosis may be accurate, but perhaps a comorbid condition was undetected or an alternate diagnosis is more appropriate. However, the treatment may be inadequate. It either may be incorrect for the condition or ineffective if prescribed at an inadequate dose. In some cases, the route of administration may be inappropriate. For example, prescribing medications taken by mouth for a patient with nausea and vomiting does not allow the drug to enter the system.

In some cases, patient noncompliance is the problem. Premature cessation of medications may be caused by side effects, fear of medications (computer research syndrome), or not following instructions. For example, medications that require a steady blood level, and must be taken daily, are often taken by the patient, "only when I think I need it." The correct medication, taken incorrectly, may lead the clinician to think it is ineffective unless the patient's compliance with instructions is confirmed.

Other confounding problems that interfere with pharmacotherapy include analgesic or caffeine overuse; conflicting medications not disclosed in the history; dietary factors; and lifestyle issues, such as poor sleep. Finally, the patient may have a poor understanding of their disorder, with greater expectations of recovery than possible. Failure to achieve the patient's expectations leads to anxiety and depression, facilitating pain. Unrealistic expectations should be addressed before treatment. What the clinician believes is a success may be seen as a failure by the patient if expectations are not discussed at the beginning of treatment.

SUMMARY

- Successful pharmacologic treatment of TMDs depends on accurate diagnosis and an understanding of the proper treatment targets.
- Acute and chronic pain, and peripheral and centralized pain, may require different pharmacologic approaches.
- Always consider what the drug does to the patient and what the patient does to the drug.

REFERENCES

1. Songer D. Psychotherapeutic approaches in the treatment of pain. Psychiatry 2005;2(5):19–24.
2. Hashmi JA, Baliki MN, Huang L, et al. Shape shifting pain: chronification of back pain shifts brain representation from nociceptive to emotional circuits. Brain 2013;136:2751–68.
3. Fletcher D. Pharmacology of anti-inflammatories and nonsteroidals. In: Beaulieu P, editor. Pharmacology of pain. Seattle: IASP Press; 2005.
4. Derry C, Derry S, Moore RA, et al. Single dose oral ibuprofen for acute postoperative pain in adults. Cochrane Database Syst Rev 2009;(3):CD001548.
5. Svensson CI, Yaksh TL. The spinal phospholipase-cyclooxygenase-prostanoid cascade in nociceptive processing. Annu Rev Pharmacol Toxicol 2002;42:553–83.
6. Högestätt ED, Jönsson BAG, Ermund A, et al. Conversion of acetaminophen to the Bioactive N-Acyl-phenolamine AM404 via fatty acid amide hydrolase-dependent arachidonic acid conjugation in the nervous system. J Biol Chem 2005;280:31405–12.
7. Pickering G, Loriot MA, Libert F, et al. Analgesic effect of acetaminophen in humans: first evidence of a central serotonergic mechanism. Clin Pharmacol Ther 2006;79(4):371–8.
8. Moore PA, Hersh EV. Combining ibuprofen and acetaminophen for acute pain management after third-molar extractions: translating clinical research to dental practice. J Am Dent Assoc 2013;144(8):898–908.
9. IASP Taxonomy - International Association for the Study of Pain. Available at: https://www.iasp-pain.org/Taxonomy. Accessed June 7, 2018.
10. Dick I, Brochu RM, Purohit Y, et al. Sodium channel blockade may contribute to the analgesic efficacy of antidepressants. J Pain 2007;8(4):315–24.
11. Lee DH, Liu X, Kim HT, et al. Receptor subtype mediating the adrenergic sensitivity of pain behavior and ectopic discharges in neuropathic Lewis rats. J Neurophysiol 1999;81:2226–33.
12. Shinder V, Govrin-Lippmann R, Cohen S, et al. Structural basis of sympathetic -sensory coupling in rat and human dorsal root ganglia following peripheral nerve injury. J Neurocytol 1999;251:1608–10.
13. Chen YW, Huang KL, Liu SY, et al. Intrathecal tricyclic antidepressants produce spinal anesthesia. Pain 2004;112:106–12.
14. Park CH, Yong A, Lee SH. Involvement of selective alpha-2 adrenoreceptor in sympathetically maintained pain. J Korean Neurosurg Soc 2010;47(6):420–3.
15. Hansson P, Leffler AS, Yarnitzky D. Pain modulation in painful neuropathy: workshop summary: endogenous pain modulation in painful neuropathy; in abstracts of the Third International Congress on Neuropathic Pain. Eur J Pain Suppl 2010;4(1):41.
16. Milanlioglu A. Paroxetine-induced severe sleep bruxism successfully treated with buspirone. Clinics (Sao Paulo) 2012;67(2):191–2.
17. Fishbain DA, Goldberg M, Robert Meagher B, et al. Male and female chronic pain patients categorized by DSM-III psychiatric diagnostic criteria. Pain 1986;26(2):181–97.
18. Gerwin RD, Dommerholt J, Shah JP. An expansion of Simons' integrated hypothesis of trigger point formation. Curr Pain Headache Rep 2004;8(6):468–75.
19. Svensson P, Graven-Nielsen T. Craniofacial muscle pain: review of mechanisms and clinical manifestations. J Orofac Pain 2001;15(2):117–45.
20. Crespo L, Wecker L, Dunaway G, et al. Brody's human pharmacology [Chapter: 12]. 5th edition. Elsevier; 2010.
21. Persaud R, Garas G, Silva S, et al. An evidence-based review of botulinum toxin (Botox) applications in non-cosmetic head and neck conditions. JRSM Short Rep 2013;4(2):10.
22. Langevin P, Peloso PM, Lowcock J, et al. Botulinum toxin for subacute/chronic neck pain. Cochrane Database Syst Rev 2011;(7):CD008626.

The Use of Botulinum Toxin for the Treatment of Myofascial Pain in the Masticatory Muscles

Daniel M. Laskin, DDS, MS

KEYWORDS

- Botulinum toxin • Myofascial pain • Masticatory muscles • Trigger points

KEY POINTS

- The mechanism by which muscle paralysis relieves myofascial pain is still unclear.
- Botulinum toxin may manage the symptoms of pain and dysfunction, but it does not treat the cause.
- There is no consensus regarding the effectiveness of botulinum toxin for treating myofascial pain.
- Botulinum toxin injections into the masticatory muscles is not free of potential complications.

Since the use of botulinum toxin (BT) for treating myofascial pain and dysfunction (MPD) in the masticatory muscles was first reported by Freund and Schwartz in 1998[1] there have been numerous clinical studies published on the subject. In considering the use of BT for this purpose there are three issues that need to be addressed: (1) what is the basis for its use, (2) does it work, and (3) are there any reasons why it should not be used?

BASIS FOR USING BOTULINUM TOXIN TO TREAT MYOFASCIAL PAIN AND DYSFUNCTION

There have been three theories proposed to explain how BT may be effective in treating MPD. Probably the most cited theory is that the pain and dysfunction is caused by masticatory muscle hyperactivity[2] and that this is relieved by paresis or paralysis of the muscle. However, electromyographic studies on the muscles of mastication in patients with MPD do not always show an increase in resting muscle activity.[3] Thus, this mechanism remains unproven.

A second proposed theory of etiology is that there is inflammation in the muscle and that the decrease in muscle activity produced by BT reduces the inflammation. This theory is based on the relief of tension-type headache, which is supposed to have an inflammatory basis, by BT injection.[4] However, there is no evidence of myositis being associated with MPD, nor does BT have an anti-inflammatory effect.

The final explanation for the action of BT relates to the elimination of trigger points in the muscle. These have been described as hyperirritable spots located in the muscle fibers. However, the areas of pain and tenderness in the masticatory muscles of patients with MPD do not have the characteristics usually described that would classify them as trigger points. Moreover, a critical evaluation of the trigger point phenomenon by Quintner and coworkers[5] suggests that existence of trigger points has no scientific basis.

The preceding analysis of the possible mechanisms by which BT could be effective in treating MPD indicate that, despite its extensive use, a scientific explanation of how muscle paralysis could

Disclosure: The author has nothing to disclose.
Department of Oral and Maxillofacial Surgery, Virginia Commonwealth University School of Dentistry, 521 North 11th Street, Richmond, VA 23298-0566, USA
E-mail address: dmlaskin@vcu.edu

Oral Maxillofacial Surg Clin N Am 30 (2018) 287–289
https://doi.org/10.1016/j.coms.2018.04.004

relieve the pain remains unclear. Recently, another action of BT in treating pain has been offered.[6] It was suggested that when injected into a painful muscle, the toxin is taken up by the peripheral terminals of the nociceptive afferent nerve fibers and this suppresses the peripheral and central release of algogenic neurotransmitters, such as glutamate or substance P, and thereby produces analgesia. Although promising, further studies are necessary to substantiate this claim.

EFFECTIVENESS OF BOTULINUM TOXIN IN TREATING MYOFASCIAL PAIN AND DYSFUNCTION

Even if the mechanism by which BT could treat MPD remains unclear, definitive proof of its effectiveness could still possibly justify its use. In a systemic literature review of BT therapy for treating MPD published in 2015, Chen and colleagues[7] found that of 124 reports only four met their criteria as randomized controlled trials. Because of the considerable variation in study methods and evaluation of results, they were not able to do a meta-analysis. Of the four studies included in their systematic review, those of Kurtoglu and colleagues[8] and von Lindern and colleagues[2] found short-term improvement in pain reduction, whereas the studies of Nixdorf and colleagues[9] and Ernberg and colleagues[10] showed no evidence of improvement. They concluded that no consensus could be reached on the therapeutic benefits of BT for treating MPD. A systematic review of the use of BT for myofascial pain syndromes in the head and neck showed similar results.[11] In four studies with 233 participants in which BT was compared with a placebo, one study showed significant improvement in pain intensity scores, whereas the other three showed no significant difference. They also concluded that there is insufficient evidence to support the use of BT for treating myofascial pain syndromes. Similar conclusions regarding the general use of BT for treating myofascial pain were reached by Gerwin[12] in his critical review of the literature. In the most recently published retrospective study on effectiveness of BT in refractory masticatory myalgia, only 30.6% of 116 patients reported significant relief of their pain.[13]

REASONS FOR NOT USING BOTULINUM TOXIN

There are many other reasons why BT should not be used routinely for treating MPD, even if its mechanism of action was understood and its efficacy was clearly established. The main reason is that it merely treats the symptoms and not the cause of the problem. Although this could be helpful in patient management, there are several potential side effects not found with other treatments for MPD that make this decision questionable. First, there are the same minor complications associated with any intramuscular injection (pain, bruising, and swelling). Then, it has been shown that some patients may develop severe, debilitating headaches that can persist for several weeks.[14] A small group of patients may also develop antibodies that prevent further effectiveness of BT, especially after receiving injections at frequent intervals.[15] Another risk of multiple injections is muscle atrophy. This has been reported to produce an hour-glass deformity in the temporalis muscle from multiple injections used to treat chronic tension headache,[16] deformity in the intrinsic muscles of the hand from intrapalmar injections to treat hyperhidrosis,[17] changes in volume of the masseter muscle and gonial angle,[13,18] and a decrease in condylar bone density.[19] The most serious complication with BT for treating MPD is the risk of developing paresis or paralysis in areas adjacent to the injection site causing difficulty in swallowing and speaking and respiratory problems.

Cost is also a factor that needs to be considered in determining the use of BT for treating myofascial pain. This not only involves the cost of the BT, but also the professional fee for treatment and follow-up, and this increases with the usual need for multiple injections. Moreover, the treatments are usually not covered by insurance because its use for this purpose is considered off-label. Although cost should not be a factor in selecting a particular treatment if it is the only effective therapy, the fact that there are less costly and less risky treatments that are equally effective argues against the routine use of BT.

SUMMARY

As noted in a policy statement of the American Association for Dental Research, ". . . unless there are specific and justifiable indications to the contrary, treatment of TMD patients initially should be based on the use of conservative, reversible and evidence-based therapeutic modalities."[20] BT does not fit this description, and current evidence for its effectiveness does not support its use for the routine treatment of MPD.

REFERENCES

1. Freund B, Schwartz M. The use of botulinum toxin for the treatment of temporomandibular disorders. Oral Health 1998;88:32–7.

2. von Lindern JJ, Niederhagen B, Bergé S, et al. Type A botulinum toxin in the treatment of chronic facial pain associated with masticatory hyperactivity. J Oral Maxillofac Surg 2003;61:774–8.

3. Intrieri RC, Jones GE, Alcorn JD. Masseter muscle hyperactivity and myofascial pain dysfunction syndrome: a relationship under stress. J Behav Med 1994;17:479–500.

4. Kocer A, Kocer E, Memisogullari R, et al. Interleukin-6 levels in tension-type headache. Clin J Pain 2010; 26(8):690–3.

5. Quintner JL, Bove GM, Cohen ML. A critical evaluation of the trigger point phenomenon [review]. Rheumatology (Oxford) 2015;54(3):392–9.

6. Moreau N, Dieb W, Descroix V, et al. Topical review: potential use of botulinum toxin in the management of painful posttraumatic trigeminal neuralgia. J Oral Facial Pain Headache 2017;51:7–18.

7. Chen Y-W, Chiu C-Y, Chen S-K, et al. Botulinum toxin therapy for temporomandibular joint disorders: a systematic review of randomized controlled trials. Int J Oral Maxillofac Surg 2015;44:1018–26.

8. Kurtoglu C, Gur OH, Kurkcu M, et al. Effect of botulinum toxin-A in myofascial pain patients with or without functional disc displacement. J Oral Maxillofac Surg 2008;66:1644–51.

9. Nixdorf DR, Heo G, Major PW. Randomized controlled trial of botulinum toxin for chronic myogenous orofacial pain. Pain 2002;99:465–73.

10. Ernberg M, Hedenberg-Magnusson B, List T, et al. Efficacy of botulinum toxin type A for the treatment of persistent myofascial TMD pain: a randomized, controlled, double-blind multicenter study. Pain 2011;152:1988–96.

11. Soares A, Andriolo RB, Atallalh AN, et al. Botulinum toxin for myofascial pain syndromes in adults. Cochrane Database Syst Rev 2012;(4):CD007533.

12. Gerwin R. Botulinum toxin treatment of myofascial pain: a critical review of the literature. Curr Pain Headache Rep 2012;16:413–22.

13. Khawaja SN, Scrivana SJ, Holland N, et al. Effectiveness, safety, and predictors of response to botulinum toxin type A in refractory masticatory myalgia: a retrospective study. J Oral Maxillofac Surg 2017; 75:2307–17.

14. Alam M, Arndt KA, Dover JS, et al. Severe, intractable headache after injection of botulinum A exotoxin: report of five cases. J Am Acad Dermatol 2002;47:62–5.

15. Dressler D. Clinical features of antibody-induced complete secondary failure of botulinum toxin therapy. Eur Neurol 2002;48:26–9.

16. Guyuron B, Rose K, Kriegler AN, et al. Hourglass deformity after botulinum toxin type A injection. Headache 2004;44:262–4.

17. Glass GE, Hussain M, Fleming AN, et al. Atrophy of the intrinsic muscles of the hand associated with the use of botulinum toxin-A injections for hyperhidrosis: a case report and review of the literature. J Plast Reconstr Aesthet Surg 2009;62:274–6.

18. Lee H-J, Kim SJ, Yu HS, et al. Repeated injections of botulinum toxin into the masseter muscle induce bony changes in human adults: longitudinal study. Korean J Orthod 2017;47:222–8.

19. Raphael KG, Tadinada A, Bradshaw JM, et al. Osteopenic consequences of botulinum toxin injections in the masticatory muscles: a pilot study. J Oral Rehabil 2014;41:555–63.

20. Greene CS. Managing patients with temporomandibular disorders: a new "standard of care". Am J Orthod Dentofacial Orthop 2010;138:3–4.

Surgical Versus Nonsurgical Management of Degenerative Joint Disease

Shravan Kumar Renapurkar, BDS, DMD

KEYWORDS

- Degenerative joint disease • TMJ arthralgia • Osteoarthritis • Osteoarthrosis

KEY POINTS

- Based on the stage of degeneration, the clinical features of degenerative joint disease include temporomandibular joint (TMJ) arthralgia, dysfunction, pain, malocclusion, facial/jaw deformity, and subsequent comorbidities.
- Early-stage disease without any malocclusion or deformity, when pain and limited function result from low-inflammatory/reactive changes, can be managed with nonsurgical modalities.
- When the disease is not amenable to nonsurgical treatment, minimally invasive procedures like arthrocentesis and arthroscopy are the first-line surgical treatments.
- In late stage, nonresponding patients, an open TMJ arthroplasty and reconstruction with an alloplastic total joint prosthesis are the options.
- The major goal of invasive surgical procedures is to improve form and function, with improvement in pain being a secondary benefit.

Degenerative joint disease (DJD) in the temporomandibular joint (TMJ) is a noninflammatory/low-inflammatory, progressive arthritic condition characterized by deterioration of the articular cartilage and subsequent changes in the underlying bone that results in debilitating pain, dysfunction, and possible deformity in end-stage disease. Both the terms osteoarthrosis and osteoarthritis have also been used to describe the clinicopathologic presentations.[1] Although some investigators differentiate these 2 terms on the basis of the presence of inflammation and joint changes, the difference is ambiguous and lacks high-level scientific support.[2] For the purpose of this article, the term degenerative joint disease (DJD) will be used to describe the condition, as endorsed in American Association of Oral and Maxillofacial Surgeons 2017 parameters of care.[3] The Diagnostic Criteria for Temporomandibular Disorders also categorizes osteoarthritis and osteoarthrosis under DJD.[4]

CLINICAL AND IMAGING PRESENTATION OF DEGENERATIVE JOINT DISEASE

The course of DJD varies from one patient to another. Patients most commonly complain of pain in the TMJ, clicking or crepitus, and limitation in mouth opening. Severe cases also can present with a malocclusion or dentofacial deformity.

The diagnosis of DJD should always be confirmed with imaging modalities. Computed tomography (CT) shows bony changes well, whereas MRI will help in assessment of disc position, structure, and joint effusion (**Fig. 1**).[5] Bony changes include surface erosion, subchondral cyst formation, condylar flattening, a "bird-beak" appearance with osteophyte formation, and loss of joint space[4] (**Fig. 2**).

It is of interest that some patients may show significant radiographic changes but are asymptomatic, whereas others show minimal radiographic changes and have significant symptoms.

Disclosure: The author has nothing to disclose.

Department of Oral and Maxillofacial Surgery, Virginia Commonwealth University School of Dentistry, Wood Building Room 311C, 520 North 12th Street, Richmond, VA 23298, USA

E-mail address: srenapurkar@vcu.edu

Oral Maxillofacial Surg Clin N Am 30 (2018) 291–297
https://doi.org/10.1016/j.coms.2018.04.005
1042-3699/18/© 2018 Elsevier Inc. All rights reserved.

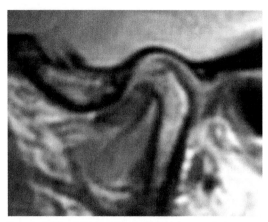

Fig. 1. MRI of TMJ with DJD and internal derangement shows anterior disc displacement and loss of the cortical outline at the superior surface of the condyle.

The diagnosis of DJD in the late stages is very straightforward based on the symptoms and articular changes, but diagnosis in the initial stages can be difficult, especially when there are few, if any, radiographic changes. Ruling out high-inflammatory arthritic conditions should also be part of the pretreatment workup. One of the commonly reported classifications for TMJ arthritis based on signs, symptoms, imaging, and management options is shown in **Table 1**.

Pathogenesis of Degenerative Joint Disease

DJD of the TMJ is a chronic condition with gradual onset and a progressive nature. The exact cause is unknown, but it is commonly associated with microtrauma or macrotrauma, joint overload, and a resultant cascade of molecular events involving the generation of free radicals, the release of proinflammatory neuropeptides and other cytokines, and then degrading enzymes.[6] This

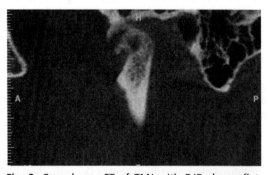

Fig. 2. Cone beam CT of TMJ with DJD shows flattening of the condylar head, "bird-beak" deformity with radiolucent "Ely" or subchondral cyst formation, and decrease of joint space.

cascade of events, combined with other contributing factors, such as age, sex, stress, medical comorbidities, hormones, diet, and so forth, creates a pathologic condition whereby the functional demands overcome the adaptive capacity of the TMJ resulting in degenerative changes. Displacement of the articular disc has also gathered significant interest as a factor that is associated with DJD.[7]

Management of Degenerative Joint Disease

The history, subjective symptoms, clinical examination findings, imaging findings, and stage of the disease should all be considered factors in determining an appropriate treatment plan. The biopsychosocial theory of TMJ dysfunction and arthralgia supports a multifactorial cause for DJD and generally encourages nonsurgical management as the primary treatment. Although DJD is considered a noninflammatory or low-inflammatory condition, secondary inflammation from the cascade of molecular events related to the pathophysiology contributes to the patient's symptoms and disease progression.[8,9] Hence, treatment of DJD aims at reducing or eliminating the inflammation and treating potential aggravating factors, thus supporting the adaptive process within the joint.

The stage of DJD plays an important role in the method of treatment selected. Early-stage DJD without significant bony changes should be treated with nonsurgical methods or minimally invasive surgical methods, such as arthrocentesis and arthroscopy, whereas late-stage disease with apertognathia and acquired mandibular retrognathia will require a combination of medical and surgical management.[1]

The role of disc position, shape, and function in the cause of DJD of the TMJ has been discussed, but a cause-effect relationship cannot be proven. Some studies report disc displacement without reduction to be an important risk factor in the progression of DJD, but it seems to be a consequence of biochemical changes in the joint rather than the cause.[10]

CURRENT EVIDENCE FOR NONSURGICAL TREATMENT OF DEGENERATIVE JOINT DISEASE

Nonsurgical methods have been recommended as the first treatment of TMJ DJD.[11] These treatments include diet modification (soft, non-chewy); behavioral/lifestyle changes; pharmacotherapy with nonsteroidal anti-inflammatory drugs (NSAIDs), muscle relaxants, antidepressants, antiepileptic agents, and corticosteroids

Table 1
Classification of temporomandibular joint arthritis based on symptoms, signs, and imaging, with management options

Stage	Symptoms	Signs	Imaging	Management Options
I. Early disease	Joint/muscle pain, limited function, crepitus	Little or no occlusal or facial esthetic changes	Mild to moderate erosive changes of condyle/fossa/eminence	Noninvasive or minimally invasive
II. Arrested disease	Little or no joint pain, muscle pain, some joint dysfunction, crepitus	Class II malocclusion, apertognathia	Flattened condyle/eminence	Bone and joint invasive or salvage
III. Advanced disease	Joint/muscle pain, loss of function ± crepitus, progressive retrognathia	High-angle class II malocclusion, apertognathia, developing fibrosis/ankylosis	Gross erosive changes, loss of condyle and eminence height, ankylosis, hypertrophy of coronoid	Salvage

From Mercuri LG. Osteoarthritis, osteoarthrosis, idiopathic condylar resorption. Oral Maxillofac Surg Clin North Am 2008;20:172; with permission.

(systemic or intra-articular); occlusal appliances; and physical therapy.

NSAIDs (Ibuprofen, Naproxen, and others) are the most commonly used pharmacotherapy for management of TMJ arthralgia because of their analgesic as well as anti-inflammatory properties[12] (see Gary M. Heir's article, "The Efficacy of Pharmacologic Treatment of Temporomandibular Disorders," in this issue). They are sometimes combined with a short tapering course of oral corticosteroid and/or with muscle relaxants to hasten the elimination or reduction of joint inflammation and decrease muscle spasm. Long-term use of NSAIDs should be viewed with caution to avoid gastrointestinal or renal toxicity.[13] Cox-2 inhibitors (Celecoxib, Meloxicam, and others) have less gastrointestinal toxicity compared with nonselective NSAIDs.[14,15] Their use in the short term has proven to be beneficial in managing TMJ pain and inflammation, but long-term use needs to be supported with level 1 studies with a large number of patients. Antidepressants and antiepileptic agents also show promising benefits in patients with temporomandibular disorder (TMD)-related arthralgia and muscle spasm, but direct benefit of these medications in arthritic conditions is not known, and use is off label.

Use of occlusal appliances in TMD has been shown to be beneficial to reduce clinical symptoms[16] (see Charles S. Greene and Harold F. Menchel's article, "The Use of Oral Appliances in the Management of Temporomandibular Disorders," in this issue). Occlusal appliances are most applicable in patients with parafunctional habits; a direct role in treatment of TMJ DJD has not been proven. These devices help in reducing the joint overload, which protects the dentition as well as helps in decreasing the muscle hyperactivity. A recent systematic review concluded that the efficacy of occlusal appliances as well as occlusal adjustments is limited and not significantly different from other modes of pain management. Hence, there is no high level evidence to support irreversible treatments, such as occlusal adjustment, to primarily manage TMJ DJD.[17] Moreover, no one appliance has been proven to be more beneficial than another.[18]

Intra-articular injections have also been used for treating DJD in the TMJ.[19–21] Hyaluronic acid (sodium hyaluronate), glucocorticosteroids, and morphine are commonly used injectable agents.[14] Narcotic agents, such as morphine and fentanyl, have a direct pain-reducing effect, but there has not been any long-term benefit or efficacy proven for such medications.

Hyaluronic acid injection is based on the theory that an impaired lubrication system contributes to the pathogenesis or progression of TMJ DJD.[20] Sodium hyaluronate mimics the synovial fluid viscosity, restores lubrication, and hampers degeneration. Although human studies show benefits in terms of pain reduction and functional improvement over the short term, and animal studies show decreased degeneration in experimentally induced arthritis, there is no evidence to show that off-label hyaluronic acid injections prevent the progression of DJD in the human TMJ.[22–24]

Glucocorticosteroid injections act by reducing the inflammation associated with the arthritic changes and hence help resolve the symptoms. Efficacy and safety of corticosteroid injections in reducing TMJ pain and improving joint function have been reported by several investigators in both short- and long-term studies.[25–28] However, there is concern for adverse effects from injection of corticosteroids into the TMJ. These adverse effects include atrophy of the adjacent skin, destruction of the cartilage, and condylar resorption. Most studies report arthropathy and condylar degeneration after multiple corticosteroid injections, but there are also a few studies in humans that show resorption after a single injection.[29–33] The factors that are involved in condylar resorption after a single use are unclear.

Physical therapy in the form of active and passive jaw exercises can help in maintaining or improving range of motion by preventing adhesions and contractures in the joint as well as by strengthening the muscles.[14,34,35] Jaw exercise can also be helpful in postsurgical patients for increasing range of motion.[36] Other therapeutic modalities, such as acupuncture, transcutaneous electrical nerve stimulation, ultrasound, and iontophoresis, have been used to help with symptoms, but their efficacy and therapeutic value are not proven by high-quality studies.[21,37]

CURRENT EVIDENCE FOR SURGICAL TREATMENT OF DEGENERATIVE JOINT DISEASE

Most patients with TMJ DJD can be managed with nonsurgical methods of treatment. Hence, surgical intervention must be based on the stage of the disease, response to noninvasive treatment, severity of dysfunction, presence of malocclusion, and/or deformity and quality-of-life issues.[38,39] Absolute indications for surgery include ankylosis, severe joint degeneration resulting in malocclusion and/or dentofacial deformity, severe pain, and loss of function (mastication). The goals of surgical intervention are to improve joint function, correct any malocclusion or deformity, prevent disability, and reduce or relieve pain. Common surgical interventions include osseous recontouring, disc repair or removal, condylotomy, orthognathic surgery, and alloplastic total joint reconstruction.

Minimally invasive surgical techniques, such as arthrocentesis and arthroscopy, are based on the principle of lysis of the adhesions, lavage of the joint to remove the inflammatory mediators, and improvement in jaw motion (see Daniel M. Laskin article, "Arthroscopy versus Arthrocentesis for Treating Internal Derangements of the Temporomandibular Joint," in this issue). Arthrocentesis is less invasive than arthroscopy and can be performed with one or 2 hypodermic needles. It also can be performed with local anesthesia and sedation or under general anesthesia, whereas arthroscopy generally requires a general anesthetic.

Nitzan and colleagues[40] reported long-term outcomes of arthrocentesis in 79 patients with TMJ osteoarthritis followed for 56.9 ± 6.7 months, with about 81% reporting favorable results. This study also showed no correlation between the outcomes and radiographic severity of the joint changes. Studies of arthrocentesis combined with injectable agents, such as hyaluronic acid or glucocorticoids, have shown little or no additional benefit.[41,42] Although arthrocentesis can be performed under local anesthesia and sedation or general anesthesia, the latter is preferable based on the ability to more adequately manipulate the jaw, increase joint mobility, and facilitate accuracy in needle placement.[43,44]

Arthroscopy, in contrast to arthrocentesis, requires elaborate equipment and is commonly performed under deep sedation or general anesthesia. The advantage arthroscopy offers is visualization of the internal joint structure, early clinical diagnosis, and correlation with the imaging findings. In addition, operative arthroscopy provides the ability to perform biopsy, discopexy, removal of adhesions and synovial plica, and other surgical manipulations. However, evidence supporting the efficacy of operative arthroscopy over lysis and lavage is limited, and most outcomes reported are similar.[45,46] The role of altered disc position in the progression of the TMJ DJD is controversial, and improvement in symptoms despite no change in the disc position does not support the assumption that it is a factor.

When minimally invasive procedures are not successful in addressing the condition, or the patient presents with end-stage DJD resulting in malocclusion and/or dentofacial deformity, open surgical interventions may be considered.

Arthroplasty is the most common operation. It involves osseous recontouring extending from a high condylar shave to a condylectomy. Although a high condylar shave (elimination of osteophytes, irregularities, erosions, and similar) has been reported to provide symptomatic relief, concern about the long-term effects of these changes on the remaining condylar segment exists.[1,47,48]

Discectomy remains one of the commonly performed procedures in patients with DJD and an internal derangement when the disc is not salvageable.[49] In such cases, its replacement remains controversial. Many autogenous and alloplastic disc replacement options have been reported. Autogenous disc replacement options include a temporalis pedicle flap, an auricular cartilage graft, and abdominal dermis-fat grafts, whereas reported alloplastic options include silicone, Proplast, and alloplastic fossa implants.[50–52] No single autogenous disc replacement option has been found to be more effective than another, nor have they been found to be superior to discectomy alone without replacement.[53] Moreover, alloplastic disc replacement materials have been largely condemned because of the foreign body reactions and the adverse effects of a metal surface against natural host tissues.[54]

Patients with severe, active, progressive condylar degenerative disease and a resultant dentofacial deformity show significant chance for relapse of the disease and the deformity when treated with orthognathic surgery alone.[55] The most predictable treatment in such conditions has been reported to be condylectomy followed by reconstruction using an alloplastic TMJ prosthesis with or without concomitant orthognathic surgery. If the degenerative changes in the TMJ are inactive in patients with Wilkes stage II-III internal derangement and a concomitant dentofacial deformity, combined TMJ arthroplasty, disc repositioning, and orthognathic surgery can be performed.[56,57]

SUMMARY

DJD is the most common condition affecting the TMJ. Because of the limited success with more aggressive interventions, the primary treatment should always be nonsurgical. Although most patients with DJD can be managed with nonsurgical modalities, those who do not respond may need minimally invasive surgical procedures, such as arthrocentesis or arthroscopy. Open surgical treatment should be reserved for those cases wherein all the previous treatments fail or end-stage DJD creates a malocclusion and/or a dentofacial deformity that requires reconstruction.

REFERENCES

1. Mercuri LG. Osteoarthritis, osteoarthrosis, idiopathic condylar resorption. Oral Maxillofac Surg Clin North Am 2008;20:169.
2. Milam SB. TMJ osteoarthritis. In: Laskin DM, Greene CS, Hylander WL, editors. Temporomandibular joint disorders: an evidence-based approach to diagnosis and treatment. Chicago: Quintessence; 2006. p. 105–24.
3. Bouloux G, Koslin M, Ness G, et al. Temporomandibular joint surgery. J Oral Maxillofac Surg 2017; 75(8S):e195–223.
4. Schiffman E, Ohrbach R, Truelove E, et al. Diagnostic criteria for temporomandibular disorders (DC/TMD) for clinical and research applications: recommendations of the International RDC/TMD Consortium Network* and orofacial pain special interest group. J Oral Facial Pain Headache 2014; 28(1):6–27.
5. Dias IM, Cordeiro PC, Devito KL, et al. Evaluation of temporomandibular joint disc displacement as a risk factor for osteoarthrosis. Int J Oral Maxillofac Surg 2016;45(3):313–7.
6. Milam S. Pathogenesis of degenerative temporomandibular joint arthritides. Odontology 2005;93:7–15.
7. Emshoff R, Rudisch A, Innerhofer K, et al. Temporomandibular joint internal derangement type III: relationship to magnetic resonance imaging findings of internal derangement and osteoarthrosis. Int J Oral Maxillofac Surg 2001;30:390–6.
8. Haskin CL, Milam SB, Cameron IL. Pathogenesis of degenerative joint disease in the human temporomandibular joint. Crit Rev Oral Biol Med 1995;6:248.
9. Tanaka E, Detamore M, Mercuri LG. Degenerative disorders of the temporomandibular joint: etiology, diagnosis and treatment. J Dent Res 2008;87:296.
10. Dimitroulis G. The prevalence of osteoarthrosis in cases of advanced internal derangement of the temporomandibular joint: a clinical, surgical and histological study. Int J Oral Maxillofac Surg 2005;34: 345–9.
11. De Leeuw R, Boering G, Stegenga B, et al. Symptoms of temporomandibular joint osteoarthrosis and internal derangement 30 years after nonsurgical treatment. Cranio 1995;13(2):81–8.
12. Dionne RA. Pharmacologic treatments for temporomandibular disorders. Oral Surg Oral Med Oral Pathol Oral Radiol Endod 1997;83(1):134–42.
13. Dionne RA. Pharmacologic approaches. In: Laskin DM, Greene CS, Hylander WL, editors. TMDs, an evidence-based approach to diagnosis and treatment. Chicago: Quintessence; 2006. p. 347–57.
14. Kopp S. Medical management of TMJ arthritis. In: Laskin DM, Greene CS, Hylander WL, editors. TMDs, an evidence-based approach to diagnosis and treatment. Chicago: Quintessence; 2006. p. 441–53.
15. Ouanounou A, Goldberg M, Haas D. Pharmacotherapy in temporomandibular disorders: a review. J Can Dental Assoc 2017;83:h7.
16. Kuttila M, Le Bell Y, Savolainen-Niemi E, et al. Efficiency of occlusal appliance therapy in secondary otalgia and temporomandibular disorders. Acta Odontol Scand 2002;60(4):248–54.
17. Forssell H, Kalso E. Application of principles of evidence-based medicine to occlusal treatment for temporomandibular disorders: are there lessons to be learned? J Orofacial Pain 2004;18(1):23–32.
18. Turp JC, Komine F, Hugger A. Efficacy of stabilization splints for the management of patients with

masticatory muscle pain: a qualitative systematic review. Clin Oral Investig 2004;8:179–95.

19. Altman RD. Intra-articular sodium hyaluronate in osteoarthritis of the knee. Semin Arthritis Rheum 2000;30:11–8.

20. Nitzan DW, Kreiner B, Zeltser B. TMJ lubrication system: its effect on the joint function, dysfunction, and treatment approach. Compend Contin Educ Dent 2004;25:437–44.

21. Tang YL, Zhu GQ, Hu L, et al. Effects of intra-articular administration of sodium hyaluronate on plasminogen activator system in temporomandibular joints with osteoarthritis. Oral Surg Oral Med Oral Pathol Oral Radiol Endod 2010;109(4):541–7.

22. Bertolami CN, Gay T, Clark GT, et al. Use of sodium hyaluronate in treating temporomandibular joint disorders: a randomized, double-blind, placebo-controlled clinical trial. J Oral Maxillofac Surg 1993;51:232–42.

23. Alpaslan GH, Alpaslan C. Efficacy of temporomandibular joint arthrocentesis with and without injection of sodium hyaluronate in treatment of internal derangements. J Oral Maxillofac Surg 2001;59:613–8.

24. Neo H, Jun-ichi I, Kurita K, et al. The effect of hyaluronic acid on experimental temporomandibular joint osteoarthrosis in sheep. J Oral Maxillofac Surg 1997;55:1114–9.

25. Kopp S, Carlsson GE, Haraldson T, et al. Long-term effect of intra-articular injections of sodium hyaluronate and corticosteroid on temporomandibular joint arthritis. J Oral Maxillofac Surg 1987;45:929.

26. Wenneberg B, Kopp S, Gröndahl H. Long-term effect of intra-articular injections of a glucocorticosteroid into the TMJ: a clinical and radiographic 8-year follow-up. J Craniomandib Disord 1991;5(1):11–8.

27. Alstergren P, Appelgren A, Appelgren B, et al. The effect on joint fluid concentration of neuropeptide Y by intra-articular injection of glucocorticoid in temporomandibular joint arthritis. Acta Odontol Scand 1996;54:1.

28. Friedman D, Moore M. The efficacy of intra-articular steroids in osteoarthritis: a double-blind study. J Rheumatol 1980;7:850–6.

29. Liu Y, Wu J, Fei W, et al. Is there a difference with intraarticular injections of corticosteroids, hyaluranate, or placebo for temporomandibular osteoarthritis? J Oral Maxillofac Surg 2018;76(3):504–14.

30. Schindler C, Paessler L, Eckelt U, et al. Severe temporomandibular dysfunction and joint destruction after intra-articular injection of triamcinolone. J Oral Pathol Med 2005;34:184.

31. Toller P. Use and misuse of intra-articular corticosteroids in the treatment of TMJ pain. Proc R Soc Med 1977;70:461–3.

32. Moskowitz R, Davis W, Sammarco J, et al. Experimentally induced corticosteroid arthropathy. Arthritis Rheum 1970;13:236–43.

33. Chandler GN, Wright V. Deleterious effect of intra-articular hydrocortisone. Lancet 1958;2:661–3.

34. Glass EG, McGlynn FD, Glaros AG. A survey of treatments for myofascial pain. Cranio 1991;9:165–8.

35. Nicolakis P, Burak EC, Kollmitzer J, et al. An investigation of the effectiveness of exercise and manual therapy in treating symptoms of TMJ osteoarthritis. Cranio 2001;19:26–32.

36. Oh DW, Kim KS, Lee GW. The effect of physiotherapy on post-temporomandibular joint surgery patients. J Oral Rehabil 2002;29:441–6.

37. List T, Axelsson S. Management of TMD: evidence from systematic reviews and meta-analyses. J Oral Rehabil 2010;37(6):430–51.

38. De Souza R, Lovato Da Silva C, Nasser M, et al. Interventions for the management of temporomandibular joint osteoarthritis. Cochrane Database Syst Rev 2012;(4):CD007261.

39. Mercuri LG. Surgical management of TMJ arthritis. In: Laskin DM, Greene CS, Hylander WL, editors. Temporomandibular joint disorders: an evidence-based approach to diagnosis and treatment. Chicago: Quintessence; 2006.

40. Nitzan DW, Svidovsky J, Zini A, et al. Effect of arthrocentesis on symptomatic osteoarthritis of the temporomandibular joint and analysis of the effect of preoperative clinical and radiologic features. J Oral Maxillofac Surg 2017;75:260–7.

41. Cömert Kiliç S. Does injection of corticosteroid after arthrocentesis improve outcomes of temporomandibular joint osteoarthritis? A randomized clinical trial. J Oral Maxillofac Surg 2016;74(11):2151–8.

42. Bouloux GF, Chou J, Krishnan D, et al. Is hyaluronic acid or corticosteroid superior to lactated ringer solution in the short-term reduction of temporomandibular joint pain after arthrocentesis? Part 1. J Oral Maxillofac Surg 2017;75(1):52–62.

43. Mehra P, Arya V. Temporomandibular joint arthrocentesis: outcomes under intravenous sedation versus general anesthesia. J Oral Maxillofac Surg 2015;73(5):834–42.

44. Tuz HH, Baslarli O, Adiloglu S, et al. Comparison of local and general anaesthesia for arthrocentesis of the temporomandibular joint. Br J Oral Maxillofac Surg 2016;54(8):946–9.

45. De La Sen Corcuera O, Cruz AM, Bascones AE, et al. Effectiveness of TMJ arthroscopy for the treatment of temporomandibular disorders, comparing lysis and lavage with operative arthroscopy. Int J Oral Maxillofac Surg 2013;42(10):1370.

46. González-García R, Rodríguez-Campo FJ. Arthroscopic lysis and lavage versus operative arthroscopy in the outcome of temporomandibular joint internal derangement: a comparative study based on wilkes stages. J Oral Maxillofac Surg 2011;69(10):2513–24.

47. Henny FA, Baldridge OL. Condylectomy for the persistently painful temporomandibular joint. J Oral Surg 1957;15:24–31.

48. Dingman RO, Grabb WC. Intra-capsular temporomandibular joint arthroplasty. Plast Reconstr Surg 1966;38:179–85.

49. Miloro M, Henriksen B. Discectomy as the primary surgical option for internal derangement of the temporomandibular joint. J Oral Maxillofac Surg 2010;68(4):782–9.

50. Bach DE, Waite PD, Adams RC. Autologous TMJ disk replacement. J Am Dent Assoc 1994;125: 1504–12.

51. Mercuri LG. Alloplastic temporomandibular reconstruction. Oral Surg 1998;85:631–7.

52. Park J, Keller EE, Reid KI. Surgical management of advanced degenerative arthritis of temporomandibular joint with metal fossa-eminence hemijoint replacement prosthesis: an 8-year retrospective survey pilot study. J Oral Maxillofac Surg 2004;62: 320–8.

53. Kramer A, Lee L, Beirne O. Meta-analysis of TMJ discectomy with or without autogenous/alloplastic interpositional materials: comparative analysis of functional outcome. Int J Oral Maxillofac Surg 2005;34:69–70.

54. Dimitroulis G. A critical review of interpositional grafts following temporomandibular joint discectomy with an overview of the dermis-fat graft. Int J Oral Maxillofac Surg 2011;40(6):561–8.

55. Wolford LM, Reiche-Fischel O, Mehra P. Changes in temporomandibular joint dysfunction after orthognathic surgery. J Oral Maxillofac Surg 2003;61(6): 655–60.

56. Catherine Z, Breton P, Bouletreau P. Management of dentoskeletal deformity due to condylar resorption: literature review. Oral Surg Oral Med Oral Pathol Oral Radiol 2016;121(2):126–32.

57. Al-Moraissi EA, Wolford LM, Perez D, et al. Does orthognathic surgery cause or cure temporomandibular disorders? A systematic review and meta-analysis. J Oral Maxillofac Surg 2017;75:1835–47.

Malocclusion as a Cause for Temporomandibular Disorders and Orthodontics as a Treatment

Bhavna Shroff, DDS, MDentSc, MPA

KEYWORDS

- Orthodontics • Occlusion • Malocclusion • Temporomandibular joint
- Temporomandibular joint disorders

KEY POINTS

- Although patients with a temporomandibular disorder (TMD) may have a malocclusion, there is no proven role for its causing the TMD, nor is there evidence for orthodontics as a cure for TMDs.
- The initial clinical examination of patients is critical in recording any preexisting TMD symptoms, referring to a TMD specialist and monitoring them during Orthodontic treatment.

INTRODUCTION

Orthodontics and temporomandibular disorders (TMDs) have been associated in the literature for many years through observations and experts' opinion. The existence of some studies showing that patients with malocclusions may have a higher prevalence of TMDs[1–4] has been at the root of the belief that there may be a cause-and-effect relationship. The fact that the TMJ and the occlusion of the teeth are anatomically related has added to the confusion. As a result of these issues, it has also been claimed that orthodontics can be a cure for TMDs.

One of the most defining events for the specialty of orthodontics was a lawsuit filed in 1987 by a patient who claimed that orthodontic treatment caused her to suffer from a TMD. To the stupefaction of the orthodontic community, the patient won the lawsuit with a large compensation, creating much anxiety concerning the orthodontist's responsibility for the onset of TMDs. This belief, still alive today, implies that TMDs can result from occlusal irregularities, and a cure for the problem is to seek alignment of the teeth into their proper position through orthodontics alone or in combination with orthognathic surgery. The goal of this article is to determine if there is evidence for this idea in the scientific literature.

MALOCCLUSION AS A CAUSE FOR TEMPOROMANDIBULAR DISORDERS AND ORTHODONTICS AS A CURE

In 1934, the otolaryngologist Costen[5] described a syndrome that hypothesized that adverse changes in the occlusion may have an effect on the TMJ, thus causing a TMD. He established this relationship after observing 11 patients whose symptoms improved following occlusal corrections involving their overbites and vertical dimension. Thus Costen syndrome was born, and the occlusion was tied to the existence of potential temporomandibular joint problems. Subsequent studies suggested that occlusal equilibration aimed at normalizing the interocclusal dental contacts would help in relief of the TMJ symptoms.[6,7]

Disclosure: The author has nothing to disclose.
Department of Orthodontics, Virginia Commonwealth University School of Dentistry, 520 North 12th Street, Suite111, Richmond, VA 23298, USA
E-mail address: bshroff@vcu.edu

Oral Maxillofacial Surg Clin N Am 30 (2018) 299–302
https://doi.org/10.1016/j.coms.2018.04.006

However, the findings in subsequent studies investigating the impact of experimental interferences on the onset of TMJ symptoms have been inconsistent and inconclusive.[8–11]

Thompson,[12] an orthodontist, in 1964 introduced the concept that malocclusions caused a displacement of the condyle posteriorly and superiorly, thus implying that correcting the dental malocclusion would favorably affect the TMD symptoms. Despite a comprehensive list of 10 myths concerning the relationship between malocclusion and TMD that was developed in the late 1980s by Greene and Laskin,[13] this association is still well and alive in the specialty of orthodontics.

McNamara,[14] in a comprehensive review of the literature in 1997, explored whether the correction of a malocclusion would influence the symptoms of a TMD. He found no difference in the occurrence of TMD symptoms in orthodontically treated and untreated patients. Although several investigators have shown that there may be a trend toward a reduction of TMD symptoms in orthodontically treated populations, most of the patients in these studies did not present with severe TMD symptoms before treatment.[14–16] The only occlusal condition that may be of significant interest when exploring the role of malocclusions and their treatment in the onset and potential treatment of TMD symptoms seems to be the presence of a unilateral crossbite. Pullinger and colleagues[15,17] suggested that an uncorrected unilateral crossbite in childhood may not always result in sufficient condylar adaptation to avoid the onset of TMD symptoms. Thilander[18] has long recommended that unilateral crossbites should be corrected at an early age to avoid asymmetric mandibular growth and unilateral condylar displacement, but the evidence supporting such practice is still debated.[19] McNamara concluded from his review of the literature that healthy patients may display increasing symptoms of a TMD during adolescence and that orthodontic treatment did not increase or decrease the odds of developing TMD symptoms at a later age.[14,20]

It has also been suggested that the type of orthodontic appliance used may be one of the potential culprits in the development of TMD symptoms. Studies conducted with either functional appliances (headgears), or fixed appliances that positioned the mandible forward, have not been conclusive on this issue.[21,22] Dibbets and colleagues[23] came to similar conclusions in a study involving 71 boys and 94 girls who presented with a variety of malocclusions (class I, class II division 1, class II division 2) and were treated with functional or fixed appliances. After great attempts to classify the TMD symptoms before the initiation of orthodontic treatment, the investigators realized that the symptoms were not consistent, but were sporadic. From this study, they concluded that the symptoms were not related to the treatment, and thus, that there was no evidence to support an association between orthodontic treatment and the appearance or persistence of TMD symptoms.[23]

Extraction of teeth for orthodontic purposes has also been blamed for increasing the incidence of TMD symptoms. Several studies have attempted to investigate this issue and have not been able to demonstrate any relationship. Sadowsky and colleagues[24] followed a cohort of 160 patients and monitored the TMD signs and symptoms before and after orthodontic treatment involving extraction of premolars. The results of the study did not show any increase in TMD symptoms after treatment involving extractions. Additional studies comparing 63 patients treated with or without extractions at the University of St Louis also did not demonstrate a difference in TMD symptoms in the 2 populations.[25,26] A long-term follow-up study of this sample of the patients concluded similarly, supporting the fact that there was no difference in the TMD symptoms with the 2 treatment modalities.[27]

Similar conclusions were reached by Dibbets and van der Weele,[28] who studied 111 patients over 15 years. A variety of treatment modalities were explored, including nonextraction (34%), extraction of premolars (29%), functional appliances (37%), and the remainder of the sample, including some fixed Begg appliance treatment and some chin cup therapy. The symptoms seemed to increase at the 4-year posttreatment evaluation and then stabilized at 10 years across the groups. After 15 years, the investigators described a slight difference for the extraction group, but they attributed the difference to growth rather than to the treatment modality. At 20 years, there was no difference between the groups, supporting other studies cited earlier.[27,28]

A recent study by Manfredini and colleagues[29] has attempted to answer some of the questions surrounding the association between a malocclusion and TMDs using a clinical trial. The central question of the study was 2-fold:

1. Is there a relationship between the presence of TMD and a history of previous orthodontic therapy?
2. Are individuals that have undergone orthodontic treatment less prone to develop a TMD when their treatment outcomes are ideal compared with those who may have a compromised nonideal result?

The researchers compared 2 groups of patients matched for age and sex. One group of patients was seeking treatment of their TMD, and the other, a control group of TMD-free patients, was seeking dental treatment. The TMD group comprised 35.1% of patients with muscle pain, 40.6% of patients with joint pain, 54% of patients with disc displacement, and 18.3% of patients with arthrosis. Extensive evaluation of the occlusal relationships, a history of prior orthodontic treatment, and assessment of the TMD were performed. They found that there was no correlation between occurrence of a TMD and a history of orthodontic treatment. In the control group, the correlation between an ideal and nonideal occlusion and the presence of a TMD also was not significant. The investigators concluded that there was no relationship between TMDs and orthodontics, and that if such relationship arose in a patient, it should be viewed as occurring by chance alone.[29]

A recent prospective study[30] questioned the role of intermaxillary class II elastics in the onset of TMD symptoms because there have been contradictory speculations in the literature supporting both a healing role of forward positioning of the mandible and its role in aggravating existing pathologic condition. Forty consecutive orthodontic patients with no TMD symptoms or previous TMD history, and treated with no extractions, were instructed to wear bilateral class II elastics full time. The patients were followed for 1 week before starting the treatment, at 24 hours, and at 1 week, and 1 month after the start of treatment. Pain was evaluated through 4 questions, and a visual analog scale was also used. Of the sample, 77.5% were female patients and 22.5% were male patients. There was pain at the onset of treatment and up to 1 week, but after a month, there was no significant difference from the baseline pain levels. The results from this study are supported by a previous study comparing 60 treated and 60 untreated patients who received extraction treatment and class II elastics.[31] No difference between the groups was reported when comparing TMD symptoms. Thus, the use of such elastics is not a potential cause for TMDs.

Luther,[32] in a 2-part review article, explored the possible association of TMDs with a functional occlusion and malocclusion. His conclusions were consistent with previous studies[8,16,33–35] that more well-controlled and well-designed studies are necessary and that the potential correlation between TMDs and a malocclusion does not mean that there is a causality effect. He also concluded that the presence of a malocclusion or its treatment with orthodontic therapy cannot be considered a cause or a cure for TMDs symptoms.[32,36] A systematic review on the relationship between TMD, malocclusion, and orthodontic treatment also investigated this controversy.[19]

The review was designed as a part of the Swedish Council on Technology Assessment in Health Care and included the literature from 1966 to 2005. The search found 58 papers that met the selection criteria, and the studies were either prospective, cohort, or retrospective. The conclusions were consistent with other studies presented in this article and supported that there is no clear association between TMDs and any specific type of malocclusion.

SUMMARY

A long history suggesting a relationship between a malocclusion and the onset of a TMD exists in the literature and has contributed to the existence of a myth that is still alive today. The abundance of case reports and low level evidence studies supporting this concept has made it challenging to establish that there is a lack of such a relationship. However, more recent well-designed clinical trials, and the modern standards of practice that use scientific evidence-based information, have made it easier to disregard the low-level evidence. These studies have clearly established that the unrelated juxtaposition of TMD symptoms and the presence of a malocclusion is at the root of the confusion and that orthodontic correction of the malocclusion will not cure the problem.

REFERENCES

1. Celic R, Jerolimov V, Panduric J. A study of influence of occlusal factors and parafunctional habits on the prevalence of signs and symptoms of TMD. Int J Prosthodont 2002;15:43–8.
2. Miller J, Burgess J, Critchlow C. Association between mandibular retrognathia and TMJ disorders in adult females. J Public Health Dent 2004;64: 157–63.
3. Egermark I, Magnusson T, Carlsson G. A 20-year follow-up of signs and symptoms of temporomandibular disorders and malocclusions in subjects with and without orthodontics and orthognathic treatment. Angle Orthod 2003;73:109–15.
4. Abrahamssson C, Henrikson T, Nilner M, et al. TMD before and after correction of dentofacial deformities by orthodontic and orthognathic treatment. Int J Oral Maxillofac Surg 2013;42:752–8.
5. Costen J. A syndrome of ear and sinus symptoms dependent upon disturbed function of the temporomandibular joint. Ann Otol Rhinol Laryngol 1934;43: 1–15.
6. Ramfjord S. Bruxism, a clinical and electromyographic study. J Am Dent Assoc 1961;62:21–44.
7. Ash M, Ramfjord S. Occlusion. 4th edition. Philadelphia: Saunders; 1995.

8. Ikeda T, Nakado M, Bando E, et al. The effect of light premature occlusal contact on tooth pain threshold in human. J Oral Rehabil 1998;25:589–95.

9. Kobayashi Y. Influences of occlusal interference on human body. J Int Coll Dent 1982;13:56–64.

10. McGlynn F, Bichajian C, Tira D, et al. The effect of experimental stress and experimental occlusal interferences on masseteric EMG activity. J Craniomandib Disord 1989;3:87–92.

11. Sheikholeslam A, Riise C. Influence of experimental interfering occlusal contacts on the activity of the anterior temporal and masseter muscles during submaximal and maximal intercuspal position. J Oral Rehabil 1983;10:207–14.

12. Thompson J. Temporomandibular disorders: diagnosis and treatment. In: Sarnat B, editor. The temporomandibular joint. 2nd edition. Springfield (IL): Charles C. Thomas; 1964. p. 146–84.

13. Greene CS, Laskin DM. Long-term status of TM clicking in patients with myofascial pain and dysfunction. J Am Dent Assoc 1988;117:461–5.

14. McNamara J. Orthodontic treatment and temporomandibular disorders. Oral Surg Oral Med Oral Pathol Oral Radiol Endod 1997;83:107–17.

15. Egermark I, Thilander B. Craniomandibular disorders with special reference to orthodontic treatment: an evaluation from childhood to adulthood. Am J Orthod Dentofacial Orthop 1992;101:28–34.

16. Magnusson T, Egermark-Eriksson I, Carlsson G. Five-year longitudinal study of signs and symptoms of mandibular dysfunction in adolescents CRANIO®. J Craniomand Pract 1996;4:338–44.

17. Pullinger A, Seligman D, Gornhein A. A multiple regression analysis of the risk and relative odds of temporomandibular disorders as a function of common occlusal features. J Dent Res 1993;72:968–79.

18. Thilander B. Treatment in the mixed dentition with special regard to the indication for orthodontic treatment. Trans Eur Orthod Soc 1975;51:141–54.

19. Molhin B, Axelsson S, Paulin G, et al. TMD in relation to malocclusion and orthodontic treatment. Angle Orthod 2007;77:542–8.

20. McNamara J, Seligman D, Okeson J. Occlusion, orthodontic treatment and temporomandibular disorders. NIH Technology Assessment Conference. Bethesda, MD,1996.

21. Janson M, Hasund A. Functional problems in orthodontic patients out of retention. Eur J Orthod 1981;3: 173–9.

22. Pancherz H. The Herbst appliance: its biological effects and clinical use. Am J Orthod 1985;87:1–20.

23. Dibbets J, van der Weele L, Uildriks A. Symptoms of of TMJ dysfunction: indicators of growth patterns? J Pedod 1985;9:265–84.

24. Sadowsky C, Theisen T, Sakols E. Orthodontic treatment and temporomandibular joint sounds: a longitudinal study. Am J Orthod Dentofacial Orthop 1991;99:441–7.

25. Paquette D, Beattie J, Johnston LJ. A long-term comparison of non-extraction and bicuspid-extraction edgewise therapy in "borderline" class II patients. Am J Orthod Dentofacial Orthop 1992; 102:1–14.

26. Beattie J, Paquette D, Johnston LJ. The functional impact of extraction and non-extraction treatments: a long-term comparison in "borderline", equally-susceptible class II patients. Am J Orthod Dentofacial Orthop 1994;105:444–9.

27. Luppanapornlarp S, Johnston LJ. The effects of premolar-extraction: a long-term comparison of outcomes in "clear-cut" extractions and non-extractions class II patients. Angle Orthod 1993;63:257–72.

28. Dibbets J, van der Weele L. Long-term effects of orthodontic treatment, including extractions, on signs and symptoms attributed to CMD. Eur J Orthod 1992;14:16–20.

29. Manfredini D, Stellini E, Gracco A, et al. Orthodontics is temporomandibular disorder-neutral. Angle Orthod 2016;86:649–54.

30. Bannwart Antunes Ortega AC, Pozza H, Franco Rocha Rodrigues LL, et al. Relationship between orthodontics and temporomandibular disorders: a prospective study. J Oral Facial Pain Headache 2016;30:134–7.

31. O'Reilly M, Rinchuse D, Close J. Class II elastics and extractions and temporomandibular disorders: a longitudinal prospective study. Am J Orthod Dentofacial Orthop 1993;103:459–63.

32. Luther F. Orthodontics and the temporomandibular joint: where are we now? Part 2. Functional occlusion, malocclusion, and TMD. Angle Orthod 1998; 68:305–18.

33. Egermark-Eriksson I, Carlsson G, Ingervall B. Prevalence of mandibular dysfunction and orofacial parafunction in 7-, 11- and 15-year-old Swedish children. Eur J Orthod 1981;3:163–72.

34. Christensen L, Rassouli N. Experimental occlusal interferences. Part I: a review. J Oral Rehabil 1995;22: 515–20.

35. Ingervall B, Carlsson G. Masticatory muscle activity before and after elimination of balancing side occlusal interference. J Oral Rehabil 1982;9:183–92.

36. Luther F. Orthodontics and temporomandibular joint: where are we now? Part 1: orthodontic treatment and temporomandibular disorders. Angle Orthod 1998;68:296–304.

Orthognathic Surgery as a Treatment for Temporomandibular Disorders

M. Franklin Dolwick, DMD, PhD[a],*,
Charles G. Widmer, DDS, MS[b]

KEYWORDS

• Orthognathic surgery • Temporomandibular disorders • Skeletal malocclusion

KEY POINTS

• The impact of orthognathic surgery on the signs and symptoms of temporomandibular disorders (TMDs) has been unclear.
• Many studies have not evaluated single jaw surgeries; instead, TMD outcomes assessments were the result of a mixture of osteotomies combined with preorthodontic and postorthodontic therapy.
• Most clinical studies on the effects of orthognathic surgery on TMD signs and symptoms did not include a control group and, when included, most control groups were not matched on age and sex.
• The best evidence in the current literature supports the concept that orthognathic surgery does not increase the overall frequency of TMD signs and symptoms at a follow-up of 2 years or more.
• However, correction of a retrognathic mandible with a counterclockwise rotation increased masticatory muscle myalgia and, combined with a 7 mm advancement, elicited an increase in myalgia and TMJ arthralgia.

INTRODUCTION

Temporomandibular disorders (TMDs) are musculoskeletal disorders involving the temporomandibular joint (TMJ), masticatory muscles, or both. Treatments for TMDs that have moderate evidence for pain reduction efficacy include pharmacologic therapies,[1–3] physical medicine,[4] behavioral therapies,[5,6] and occlusal appliance therapies.[7,8] These treatment approaches are considered reversible compared with irreversible treatments, which include occlusal equilibration, mandibular repositioning, orthodontics, and orthognathic surgery.[9] In recent years, there have been reports describing early irreversible interventions such as the bilateral sagittal split osteotomy or the intraoral vertical ramus osteotomy to address skeletal malocclusions in patients with TMDs.[10] The rationale for pursuing an early surgical approach has been the clinical impression of success in reducing signs and symptoms of TMDs while correcting the skeletal malocclusion.

Clinical impressions of success are prone to different biases that can influence the perception of clinicians. For many years, these clinical impressions have driven the course of various treatments for TMDs, with the conclusion that the specified intervention was the cause for success in reducing or eliminating TMD pain and dysfunction.[11,12] In the case of orthognathic surgery, some surgeons consider their treatment to be successful in permanently resolving both a skeletal abnormality as well as a musculoskeletal disorder, particularly one associated with pain.[13] To address this question,

Disclosure: The authors have nothing to disclose.
[a] Department of Oral and Maxillofacial Surgery, University of Florida College of Dentistry, PO Box 100416, Gainesville, FL 32610-0416, USA; [b] Division of Facial Pain, Department of Orthodontics, University of Florida College of Dentistry, PO Box 100444, Gainesville, FL 32610-0444, USA
* Corresponding author.
E-mail address: fdolwick@dental.ufl.edu

Oral Maxillofacial Surg Clin N Am 30 (2018) 303–323
https://doi.org/10.1016/j.coms.2018.04.007
1042-3699/18/© 2018 Elsevier Inc. All rights reserved.

a few publications have pursued a meta-analysis of clinical studies based on well-defined inclusion and exclusion criteria.[14,15] However, there were few well-controlled studies available in the literature that addressed a specific skeletal malocclusion and allowed an adequate assessment of the outcome of orthognathic surgery on TMD.

The purpose of this article is to provide an update on the efficacy of orthognathic surgery as a treatment of TMD. This update was accomplished by assessing peer-reviewed, published studies of orthognathic surgery procedures that were performed in the absence and presence of TMD signs and symptoms. This topic has been a focus by a few previous investigators who provided an overview of their study design and target study populations. However, this review evaluates the methodology that was used to minimize observer bias (if any) and to provide an updated evidence-based assessment. It targets 3 types of skeletal malocclusions commonly addressed by orthognathic surgery: class II, class III, and anterior open bite. In addition, the surgical approach is considered as an independent variable when the results for each type of surgery are reported in the publication. Individual case studies (n = 5 or less) and meta-analyses were not included in the literature that was reviewed.

EXPERIMENTAL DESIGN OF CLINICAL STUDIES

Clinical studies that evaluated TMD signs and symptoms after orthognathic surgery were evaluated using the criteria listed in the headers of **Table 1**. These criteria were identified as important to document the quality of the experimental design and appropriateness of the statistical analyses used in the study. Fulfillment of these criteria generally ranked the study into an upper level and was viewed as contributory to the evidence that did or did not show efficacy of the orthognathic surgery as a treatment of TMDs.

Many of the reviewed studies were retrospective and commonly were consecutive cases seen at an educational institution. Retrospective studies, although convenient, have some advantages but also many limitations in providing an accurate assessment of treatment efficacy (**Table 2**). Assessing the unbiased, accurate pain outcome measures of TMDs in orthognathic surgery patients to determine the effect of this treatment requires special attention to the experimental design. It has been elegantly shown in 1 well-controlled clinical trial on migraine headaches that pain can be influenced by multiple factors, including patient expectation,[48] a factor that would be associated with any treatment approach.

Therefore, it is paramount to consider only the best evidence available to determine the effects, if any, that orthognathic surgery may have on different skeletal malocclusion types.

Retrospective studies using chart reviews also have been shown to be limited in the comprehensive review of TMD signs and symptoms compared with prospective studies.[49] Multiple signs and symptoms are frequently not included in chart documentation and the lack of these data may result in a low estimation of TMD prevalence. Thus, chart reviews should be considered a limited and potentially biased source of data to assess signs and symptoms of TMD in a clinical sample.

In many studies, the patient samples contained a mixture of skeletal malocclusion types and the proportion of subtypes was usually reported. However, the TMD outcomes associated with a specific malocclusion were commonly not reported. Instead, the entire surgical sample was evaluated for efficacy in reducing (or increasing) TMD signs and symptoms. In a few studies, there was a focus on a single malocclusion (class II, class III, or anterior open bite) rather than a group of malocclusion types and this allowed a better assessment of the effects of the surgery on masticatory musculoskeletal pain and dysfunction. These studies are discussed in greater detail later.

A few studies focused on the technique of mandibular stabilization after surgery and also evaluated TMD signs and symptoms.[28,45] One well-controlled study that randomized patients into nonrigid or rigid fixation of the mandible after a bilateral sagittal split osteotomy (BSSO) found no statistically significant difference in TMD signs and symptoms after a 2-year follow-up.[28] This study was well designed, with randomization of a relatively homogenous sample of orthognathic patients into 2 mandibular fixation groups after the patients were screened based on specific inclusion and exclusion criteria. In addition, this study used well-defined and validated TMD assay measures and calibrated examiners. The only limitation with this study, and this was acknowledged by the investigators, was the inability to minimize bias by blinding the examiners to the type of mandibular fixation. The study had sufficient statistical power to determine differences between the two groups, and none was found, so it is doubtful that the lack of blinded examiners had an impact on the study outcome measures, particularly for TMD assessment.

Random assignment of a homogenous group of orthognathic surgery patients into an experimental and a control group is an optimal experimental design but is not feasible in a clinical study of patients who are having orthognathic surgery to correct their

Table 1

Class II, class III, and anterior open-bite skeletal malocclusions: temporomandibular disorder signs and symptoms before and after orthognathic surgery

Reference	Type of Study	No. of Patients (F:M)	Surgical Approach (% Combined Ortho/Surgery)	Randomized Study/Control Group (Yes/No)	Calibrated/ Blinded Examiners (Yes/No)	Well-Defined Inclusion/ Exclusion Criteria (Yes/No)	TMD Assessment	Postsurgical Follow-up Duration	Comment
Upton et al,[16] 1984 Res. design assessment: 9	Retrospective case series	Class II: 46 (36:10) Class III: 39 (22:17) Ant. open bite: 14 (9:5)	Ortho/surgery (75%) or surgery only	No/no	No/no	No	Questionnaire	Not reported	Primary outcome variable: TMJ pain/dysfunction. Descriptive statistics reported. Inferential statistical tests not calculated for presurgical and postsurgical outcomes
Karabouta & Martis,[17] 1985 Res. design assessment: 17	Retrospective case series	Class II: 46 Class III: 161 Ant. open bite: 45	Surgery only: BSSO	No/no	No/no	No	Physical examination: TMJ pain, myofascial pain, TMJ sounds, restricted jaw movement	6 mo	Primary outcome variable: TMJ pain/dysfunction. Descriptive statistics reported. Inferential statistical tests not calculated for presurgical and postsurgical outcomes
Timmis et al,[18] 1986 Res. design assessment: 20	Prospective cohort	Class II: 25 (12 R; 13 NR) Class III: 3	Ortho/surgery: BSSO	No/no	No/no	No	Physical examination: TMJ sounds, myofascial pain, deviation with jaw opening	NR: 6–36 mo R: 6–12 mo	Primary outcome variable: TMJ pain/dysfunction incidence in R and NR fixation. No significant difference between preoperative and postoperative muscle or TMJ pain incidence. Individual skeletal malocclusion groups not statistically tested

(continued on next page)

Table 1 *(continued)*

Reference	Type of Study	No. of Patients (F:M)	Surgical Approach (% Combined Ortho/Surgery)	Randomized Study/Control Group (Yes/No)	Calibrated/Blinded Examiners (Yes/No)	Well-Defined Inclusion/Exclusion Criteria (Yes/No)	TMD Assessment	Postsurgical Follow-up Duration	Comment
Magnusson et al,[19] 1986 Res. design assessment: 17	Retrospective case series	Class II: 3 Class III: 12 Ant. open bite: 1	Ortho/surgery (65%) or surgery only: BSSO, segmental osteotomy of mandible, Le Fort I, or combination	No/no	No/no	No	Helkimo index	Variable: 1–2.5 y	Primary outcome variable: TMJ pain/dysfunction. Descriptive statistics reported. Ai significantly reduced postsurgically compared with presurgical assessments. Individual skeletal malocclusion groups not statistically tested
Kerstens et al,[20] 1989 Res. design assessment: 17	Retrospective case series	Class II: 338 Class III: 142	Ortho/surgery (91%) or surgery only: BSSO ± Le Fort I osteotomy	No/no	No/no	No	Questionnaire and physical examination (TMJ sounds, limited mandibular movement, palpable muscle tenderness)	Clinical examination: 1 y Questionnaire: 1.4–4.7 y	Primary outcome variable: TMJ pain/dysfunction. Descriptive statistics reported. No statistical difference between clinical preoperative and postoperative TMD signs or symptoms or questionnaire symptoms
Smith et al,[21] 1992 Res. design assessment: 21	Prospective cohort	Class II: 22 (14:8)	Ortho/surgery (100%): BSSO (R)	No/no	No/no	No	Modified Helkimo index	6–7 mo	Primary outcome variable: TMJ pain/dysfunction. Descriptive statistics reported. Inferential statistical tests not calculated for presurgical and postsurgical outcomes
Athanasiou & Melsen,[22] 1992 Res. design assessment: 24	Retrospective case series	Class III: 36 (25:11)	Ortho/surgery (100%): IVRO NR: 18 No fixation: 18	No/no	No/Yes	No	Modified Helkimo index Clinical examination (TMJ sounds, muscle and joint palpation, mandibular movement, ROM)	6 mo	Primary outcome variable: TMJ pain/dysfunction incidence in R and NR fixation. Maximal interincisal opening was significantly reduced by 5.4 mm. Muscle pain frequency and lateral excursive movements did not change. No statistical difference between TMD frequency in men and women

Study	Design	Patients	Intervention				Assessment	Follow-up	Outcome
De Clercq et al,[23] 1995 Res. design assessment: 15	Retrospective case series	Class II: 196 (150:46)	Surgery only: BSSO (R) ± Le Fort I osteotomy	No/no	No/no	Yes	Physical examination (muscle tenderness, joint sounds, pain, limitation of movement)	Minimum 6 mo	Primary outcome variable: TMJ pain/dysfunction. Descriptive statistics reported. Statistical decrease of TMD from 27% (preoperative) to 18% (postoperative) for all patients and from 30% (preoperative) to 1.8% (postoperative) for the normal/low angle deficiency group. No statistical difference for TMD in the high angle deficiency group
Feinerman & Piecuch,[24] 1995 Res. design assessment: 14	Retrospective case series	66 NR (21:11) R (21:13) Class II and class III patient distribution not reported	Surgery only: BSSO ± Le Fort I osteotomy (34 R, 32 NR)	No/no	No/no	No	Questionnaire and physical examination (TMJ sounds, limited jaw movement, palpable muscle or joint pain)	Variable: 2–10 y	Primary outcome variable: TMJ pain/dysfunction incidence in R and NR fixation. Descriptive statistics reported. Specific TMD outcomes not reported for class II and class III patients. Statistical differences were observed between R and NR fixation for palpable muscle tenderness (increased in NR) and TMJ clicking (increased in NR)
Onizawa et al,[25] 1995 Res. design assessment: 17	Retrospective case series	30 (20:10) class II: 10 Class III: 17	Surgery only: BSSO ± Le Fort I osteotomy	No/yes Control group: 30 dental students (11 F:19 M)	No/no	No	Questionnaire and physical examination (TMJ sounds, limited jaw movement, palpable muscle or joint pain)	6 mo	Statistically significant decreases in maximal mandibular opening and protrusion between presurgical and postsurgical assessments for class II and class III patients. No statistically significant difference between patients and controls for TMJ sounds, mandibular deviation or palpable muscle tenderness

(continued on next page)

Table 1
(continued)

Reference	Type of Study	No. of Patients (F:M)	Surgical Approach (% Combined Ortho/Surgery)	Randomized Study/Control Group (Yes/No)	Calibrated/ Blinded Examiners (Yes/No)	Well-Defined Inclusion/ Exclusion Criteria (Yes/No)	TMD Assessment	Postsurgical Follow-up Duration	Comment
Rodrigues-Garcia et al,[26] 1998 Res. design assessment: 38	Prospective cohort	Class II: 124 (92:32)	Ortho/surgery (100%): BSSO	Yes/no	Yes/no	Yes	Craniomandibular index	2 y	MI had small, statistically significant improvement after surgery. Opening clicking incidence was significantly reduced, whereas crepitus was significantly increased
Panula et al,[27] 2000 Res. design assessment: 21	Retrospective case series	60 (49:11) Class II: 49 Class III: 11	Ortho/surgery (100%): BSSO ± Le Fort I osteotomy	No/yes Control group: 20 patients who decided not to have ortho/surgery (16 F:4 M)	No/no	No	Helkimo index	Variable: 20–44 mo postsurgery	Specific TMD outcomes not reported for skeletal malocclusion subgroups (aggregate of class II, III, and ant. open bite). Statistically significant decrease of TMJ crepitus, palpable muscle and joint pain, and headaches was found. No statistically significant differences between ortho/surgery group and control group at start of study. No statistically significant differences for control group assessment at presurgery and postsurgery time points
Nemeth et al,[28] 2000 Res. design assessment: 38	Prospective cohort	64 R (47:17) 63 NR (48:15) Class II: 127 (95:32)	Ortho/surgery (100%): BSSO	Yes/no	Yes/no	Yes	CM	2 y	No statistically significant difference for overall CMI, MI, DI, or joint sounds were found between R and NR fixation
Egermark, et al,[29] 2000 Res. design assessment: 14	Retrospective case series	52 (34:18)	Ortho/surgery (100%): BSSO ± Le Fort I osteotomy	No/no	No/no	No	Modified Helkimo index	2.2–9.5 y	No description of malocclusion types. No significant differences for TMD signs and symptoms between presurgery and postsurgery outcomes

Study	Study design	Sample	Ortho/surgery				Physical examination	Follow-up	Primary outcome measures
Kobayashi et al,[30] 2000 Res. design assessment: 17	Retrospective case series	145 (99:46) Class III malocclusion ± anterior open bite	Ortho/surgery (100%): BSSO (40 R, 105 NR)	No/no	No/no	No	Physical examination (TMJ pain, sounds, movements and limitations)	1 y	Primary outcome measures: NR and R fixation relapse and TMJ pain/dysfunction. No statistically significant difference was found for relapse between R and NR fixation. No significance differences were found for TMJ pain and dysfunction between fixation groups
Westermark et al,[31] 2001 Res. design assessment: 19	Retrospective case series	1516 (958:558) Class II: 526 Class III: 580 Ant. open bite: 396	Surgery only: BSSO (R and NR) IVRO	No/no	No/no	No	Questionnaire (TMJ noise, pain, headaches, bruxism) Clinical examination (only at 2-y follow-up) 3 fingers: normal 2–3 fingers: reduced 1–2 fingers: severely reduced	2 y	Questionnaire required an accurate memory of presurgical conditions. Physical examination did not include specific measurements. Statistically significant difference for preoperative symptom-free prognathic patients developing TMD (17%) compared with symptom-free retrognathic patients developing TMD (25%)
Aghabeigi et al,[32] 2001 Res. design assessment: 17	Retrospective case series	Ant. open bite: 83 (2:1 ratio)	Ortho/surgery (100%): Le Fort I ± BSSO or IVRO osteotomy	No/no	No/no	No	Clinical examination included mandibular ROM and deviation, TMJ sounds, and TMJ and masticatory muscle pain. Questionnaire completed by 42% of patients included TMJ scale, SCL-90, STAI, and VAS for overall satisfaction	>1 y	No statistically significant difference between presurgical and postsurgical TMD assessments. Postsurgical pain was significantly associated with an abnormal psychological profile (higher stress and trait anxiety) and gender (female)

(continued on next page)

Table 1
(continued)

Reference	Type of Study	No. of Patients (F:M)	Surgical Approach (% Combined Ortho/Surgery)	Randomized Study/Control Group (Yes/No)	Calibrated/ Blinded Examiners (Yes/No)	Well-Defined Inclusion/ Exclusion Criteria (Yes/No)	TMD Assessment	Postsurgical Follow-up Duration	Comment
Dervis & Tuncer,[33] 2002 Res. design assessment: 34	Prospective cohort	50 NR (29:21) Unknown number of patients in class I, II, and III subgroups	Surgery only: BSSO ± Le Fort I osteotomy	No/yes Control group: 50 healthy subjects without TMD (28 F:22 M)	No/no	Yes	Helkimo index	2 y	No statistically significant differences between patients and controls before surgery. No significant differences found among class I, II, or III presurgical and postsurgical TMD signs or symptoms for each surgical technique (because of small N). After 2 y postoperative, significant decreases found for muscle palpation scores, Di and Ai scores in patient group. A statistically significant sex difference was found with 47% of women having improved subjective symptoms compared with 18% of men
Ueki et al,[34] 2002 Res. design assessment: 19	Retrospective case series	Class III: 43	Ortho/surgery: (100%) BSSO ± Le Fort I osteotomy (23); IVRO (20) ± Le Fort I osteotomy	No/no	No/no	No	TMJ sounds and pain with mandibular opening	6 mo	Primary outcome measures: TMJ pain/dysfunction, condylar position, anterior disc displacement. No statistically significant differences in TMJ sounds or pain between 2 surgical procedures. IVRO was associated with normalized disc position

Study	N (sex) Class	Surgery				Outcome measure	Follow-up	Results
Wolford et al,[35] 2003 Res. design assessment: 19	25 (23:2) Class II: 24	Surgery only: BSSO + Le Fort I osteotomy	No/no	No/no	Yes	Pain VAS; physical examination	Variable: 12–81 mo	TMJ pain VAS increased significantly between presurgical and postsurgical measures. Maximum mandibular vertical ROM was significantly decreased. TMJ sound changes were not statistically evaluated and reported
Pahkala & Heino,[36] 2004 Res. design assessment: 21	72 (49:23) Class II: 46 Class III: 14 Ant. open bite: 4	Ortho/surgery: (100%) BSSO (R)	No/no	No/no	No	Modified Helkimo index; AAOP TMD subgroups	Variable: mean 1.9 y (SD, 0.5)	TMJ clicking, TMJ pain, and headaches were significantly decreased (includes all skeletal malocclusion groups). Myogenous and myogenous/arthrogenous groups had significant reduction in symptoms. Arthrogenous group had no significant preoperative and postoperative differences in symptoms
Borstlap et al,[37] 2004 Res. design assessment: 31	Class II: 222 (169:53)	Ortho/surgery: (100%) BSSO (R)	No/no	No/no	Yes	Questionnaire and physical examination (TMJ sounds, limited jaw movement, palpable joint pain)	24 mo	TMJ pain was significantly decreased after 2 y, whereas clicking was unchanged compared with presurgical assessments. Maximum mandibular opening was not significantly different, whereas lateral and protrusive movements had a statistically significant decrease
Kallela et al,[38] 2005 Res. design assessment: 27	Class II: 40 (29:11)	Ortho/surgery: (100%) BSSO (R)	No/no	No/no	No	Helkimo index	Variable: 1–5 y	TMJ clicking, crepitus and muscular pain were statistically reduced postoperatively compared with preoperative assessment

(continued on next page)

Table 1
(continued)

Reference	Type of Study	No. of Patients (F:M)	Surgical Approach (% Combined Ortho/Surgery)	Randomized Study/Control Group (Yes/No)	Calibrated/ Blinded Examiners (Yes/No)	Well-Defined Inclusion/ Exclusion Criteria (Yes/No)	TMD Assessment	Postsurgical Follow-up Duration	Comment
Farella et al,[39] 2007 Res. design assessment: 33	Prospective cohort	Class III: 14 (9:5)	Ortho/surgery: (100%) BSSO (R) + Le Fort I osteotomy	No/no	No/no	Yes	Axis I of RDC for TMD and masticatory muscle PPT thresholds	12 mo	No statistically significant differences in TMJ clicking, lateral or protrusive movement, or muscle PPT assessment. A significant reduction in maximal interincisal opening was found (~5 mm)
Valle-Corotti et al,[40] 2007 Res. design assessment: 20	Prospective cohort	Class III: 25	Ortho/surgery: (100%) Unknown surgery	No/yes Control group: 25 patients only treated by orthodontics	No/no	No	Questionnaire and physical examination (TMJ sounds, limited jaw movement, palpable joint and muscle pain)	> 1 y	No statistically significant differences were found between experimental and control groups between presurgery and postsurgery or preorthodontic and postorthodontic treatment
Frey et al,[41] 2008 Res. design assessment: 40	Prospective cohort	127 (95:32) Class II: 127	Ortho/surgery (100%): BSSO Study compared amount of mandibular advancement and counterclockwise rotation	Yes/no	Yes/no	Yes	CMI	2 y	Patients who had a counterclockwise mandibular rotation had significantly more muscle symptoms. Patients who had a mandibular advancement >7 mm and a counterclockwise rotation had significantly more muscle and TMJ symptoms than shorter advancement and/or clockwise rotation

Dujoncquoy et al,[42] 2010 Res. design assessment: 13	Retrospective case series	57 (35:22)	Ortho/surgery: (100%) BSSO (R) ± Le Fort I osteotomy	No/no	No/no	Yes
Abrahamson et al,[43] 2013 Res. design assessment: 37	Retrospective case series	98 (60:38) Class II: 27 Class III: 58 Ant. open bite: 13	Ortho/surgery: (100%) BSSO, IVRO, Le Fort I, maxillary segmental osteotomies (R)	No/yes Control group: 38 healthy age-matched and sex-matched subjects without TMD	Yes/yes	Yes

Questionnaire	Variable: 6–30 mo
	Descriptive statistics reported. Inferential statistical analyses were not calculated for presurgical and postsurgical outcomes. Data were dependent on recall of TMD signs/symptoms. Results included all skeletal malocclusion groups so no assessment of impact on each skeletal malocclusion
Questionnaire and RDC for TMD physical examination (sounds, limited movement, palpable muscle pain)	36 mo
	Class III patients had a significant decrease in myofascial pain and arthralgia postsurgery. Class II patients had no significant differences in TMD signs or symptoms between presurgical and postsurgical assessment. No significant differences in mandibular mobility. Significant sex difference in myofascial pain frequency at baseline for all groups (F, 32% > M, 12%) but not postsurgery. Statistically significant decreases in frequency were found for myofascial pain, disc displacement, and arthralgia between presurgery and postsurgery for all skeletal malocclusion groups. Significant differences between patients and controls were found for myofascial pain and arthralgia for all groups

(continued on next page)

Table 1
(continued)

Reference	Type of Study	No. of Patients (F:M)	Surgical Approach (% Combined Ortho/Surgery)	Randomized Study/Control Group (Yes/No)	Calibrated/ Blinded Examiners (Yes/No)	Well-Defined Inclusion/ Exclusion Criteria (Yes/No)	TMD Assessment	Postsurgical Follow-up Duration	Comment
Togashi et al,[44] 2013 Res. design assessment: 19	Retrospective case series	170 (133:37) Class II: 20 (17:3) Class III: 131 (99:32)	Ortho/surgery: (100%) BSSO (R) ± Le Fort I osteotomy	No/no	No/no	No	Physical examination (sounds, limited movement, palpable TMJ pain)	1 y	Significant difference found for TMD signs and symptoms among skeletal malocclusion groups (prognathism, 17%; retrognathism, 40%; asymmetry, 58%). After surgery, no significant differences in signs and symptoms of TMD between subgroups. After preoperative orthodontics, no significant differences of TMD signs and symptoms compared with baseline for all orthognathic surgery patients. However, after orthognathic surgery, significant decreases of TMD signs and symptoms were found for all orthognathic surgery patients
Mladenovic et al,[45] 2013 Res. design assessment: 27	Retrospective case series	Class III: 40 (25:15)	Ortho/surgery: (100%) (25 R, 25 NR) BSSO	No/yes Control group: 42 (17:25) untreated class III patients	No/no	No	RDC for TMD	12 mo	Only statistical comparison was made postsurgery compared with controls. Prevalence of myofascial pain was similar in men and women of control group but was significantly higher in women in orthognathic surgery group, whereas TMJ pain was lower

Scolozzi et al,[46] 2015 Res. design assessment: 27	Retrospective case series	219 (123:96) Class II: 76 Class III: 51 Ant. open bite: 42	Ortho/surgery: (100%) BSSO (R) ± Le Fort I osteotomy	No/no	No/no	No	Helkimo index RDC for TMD diagnostic classification	1 y	TMJ clicking (Ai) was predictive for TMD (OR, 3.61) or MPD (OR, 2.43). TMJ clicking determined by Di, combined with Le Fort I and BSSO, statistically significant for postoperative TMD as determined by Ai. Palpable muscle tenderness was predictive of postoperative TMD (Di). Maximum mandibular opening and mandibular protrusion were significantly decreased postsurgery and mandibular deviation was increased
Yoon et al,[10] 2015 Res. design assessment: 29	Retrospective case series	30 (11:4) Class III: 30	Surgery only: BSSO (R) + Le Fort I osteotomy	No/yes Control group: 15 (8:7) class III, 2 jaw surgery and TMD treatment	No/no	Yes	Questionnaire (subjective changes in TMD symptoms) and RDC for TMD clinical examination (ROM <35 mm, TMJ sounds, TMJ pain)	6 mo or more	Both experimental and control groups had class III skeletal malocclusion and TMD signs and symptoms before surgery. Experimental group (surgical group) had no prior TMD treatment and had a statistically significant reduction in TMJ noise and pain after surgery. The control group had treatment of TMD until signs/symptoms were eliminated before surgery and had a significant reduction in TMJ noise but not pain

(continued on next page)

Table 1
(continued)

Reference	Type of Study	No. of Patients (F:M)	Surgical Approach (% Combined Ortho/Surgery)	Randomized Study/Control Group (Yes/No)	Calibrated/ Blinded Examiners (Yes/No)	Well-Defined Inclusion/ Exclusion Criteria (Yes/No)	TMD Assessment	Postsurgical Follow-up Duration	Comment
Sebastiani et al,[13] 2016 Res. design assessment: 25	Prospective cohort	54 Class I: 4 Class II: 17 Class III: 33	Surgery only: BSSO (R) ± Le Fort I osteotomy	No/no	No/no	Yes	RDC for TMD; (TMJ sounds, muscle or TMJ pain, mandibular mobility)	6 mo	Specific TMD outcomes not reported for class I, II, and III patients. Inappropriate statistical tests (univariate tests) were used when comparing 3 or more variables. Overall, a significant decrease TMJ sounds was reported comparing preoperative and postoperative assessments. No statistically significant changes were noted for arthralgia, muscle pain, or maximum opening with pain. A significant difference was found between preoperative and postoperative maximum mandibular opening without pain
Di Paolo et al,[47] 2017 Res. design assessment: 17	Retrospective case series	76 Malocclusion types and frequency not reported	Ortho/surgery: (100%) BSSO (R) ± Le Fort I osteotomy	No/no	No/no	Yes	RDC for TMD; (TMJ sounds, muscle or TMJ pain, mandibular mobility)	6–12 mo	Statistical differences for presurgery and postsurgery outcomes were not clearly reported

Abbreviations: AAOP, American Academy of Orofacial Pain; Ai, anamnestic index of Helkimo; Ant., anterior; BSSO, bilateral sagittal split osteotomy; CMI, craniomandibular index; Di, clinical dysfunction index of Helkimo; DI, dysfunction index, a subindex of the CMI; F, female; IVRO: intraoral vertical ramus osteotomy; M, male; MI, muscle index, a subindex of the CMI; MPD, myofascial pain dysfunction; N, number of patients in study; NR, nonrigid fixation; OR, odds ratio; PPT, pressure pain threshold; R, rigid fixation; RDC, research diagnostic criteria; Res., research; ROM, range of motion; SCL-90, symptom checklist-90; SD, standard deviation; STAI, Spielberger state–trait anxiety inventory; TMD, temporomandibular disorders; VAS, visual analog scale.

Table 2
Advantages and limitations of a retrospective study for a pain condition

Advantages	Limitations
• Has the potential to collect data from a large number of patients • Retrospective chart reviews are relatively inexpensive • Can provide some limited information on the characteristics of a study sample and their response to treatment • Can be valuable in rare pain conditions in which the number of patients is low and there is a paucity of treatment outcome assessment • Can provide data to generate hypotheses for a prospective pain study	• Missing data are a limitation because there usually is not a standardized set of data acquisition variables that are complete for all patients • Limited or no inclusion and exclusion criteria to identify a homogenous group of patients • Patients are not randomly selected (usually referrals) and may not represent the general population • Lack of a parallel control group matched for age/sex/ethnicity • Some retrospective studies require patients to recall their pain conditions after months/years and there is good evidence that memory of pain is not accurate • Lack of methods to calibrate a single examiner or multiple examiners to minimize examiner bias • Lack of blinded examiners to minimize examiner bias • Descriptive statistical reporting is common but inferential statistical testing is often not conducted or is limited by an inadequate sample size when stratification of patients is performed (ie, sex, age, type of malocclusion, type of surgery)

malocclusion. However, control groups were incorporated into some studies.[10,25,27,33,40,43,45] They consisted of non-patients with TMD such as dental students, orthodontic patients who did not want to pursue orthognathic surgery, or untreated patients with the same malocclusion as the experimental orthognathic surgery patients. Some studies matched the control patients by age and sex, whereas other studies did not incorporate this requirement in their control patients. Using unmatched controls is a major flaw in TMD studies because sex and age are two known factors that have an impact on the prevalence of TMD signs and symptoms.

INFLUENCE OF ORTHODONTIC TREATMENT

Most patients in the reviewed studies (25 out of 34, or 74%) had orthodontic treatment before orthognathic surgery, which is a potential confounding factor because it is possible that the signs and symptoms of patients with TMD could be greater at the orthodontic assessment time and could spontaneously be reduced during the treatment period. This issue was examined by de Boever and colleagues,[50] who reported no statistically significant differences between T1 and T2 time points

(preorthodontics and presurgery) in a subgroup of 30 patients in their study. However, this subgroup was probably statistically underpowered because of the small N (number of patients in study). Support for this criticism is based on publication of a similar study that found statistically significant differences over time for the muscle index only after combining the groups to increase the number of patients.[41] One consideration for future studies would be to have a parallel age-matched and sex-matched control group similar to the orthognathic surgery group that was pursuing orthodontic therapy and to continue to evaluate both groups over time using the same assay time points. Using this strategy, combined with control of experimental bias, it would be possible to more accurately determine the effect that orthognathic surgery may have on TMD signs and symptoms.

CONTROL OF EXPERIMENTAL BIAS

Experimental biases can appear in many different aspects of a clinical study and can be seen in most of the reviewed studies. Well-designed randomized clinical trials require a rigorous attempt to minimize various sources of bias, but this cannot be achieved in retrospective studies because of the lack of preplanned experimental design and data acquisition. Examples of different experimental biases that were observed in the reviewed literature are shown in **Table 3**.

Another form of bias that has received more recent attention is the manipulation of acquired data, statistical analysis, and output bias.[51] It is unknown whether any orthognathic surgery clinical studies that were reviewed had such bias because none were registered in ClinicalTrials.gov to allow a comparison of the proposed experimental design and the reported outcomes measures in the publications. However, registered neurology clinical trials were found to have 66% major discrepancies in the experimental design and statistical reporting (eg, primary and secondary outcome variables switched; timing of data collection; discrepancies in reporting of probability values).

ASSESSMENT OF BIAS MINIMIZATION IN ORTHOGNATHIC SURGERY CLINICAL STUDIES

Assessment of clinical studies that evaluated orthognathic surgery for TMD management based on specific research design criteria would be an objective method to determine the relative impact of one published study relative to other published studies. Therefore, a criteria-based assessment was developed (**Table 4**) and applied to each clinical study that was reviewed (reported in column 1 in **Table 1**). The distribution of assessment scores ranged from 9 to 40 and had a bimodal distribution (**Fig. 1**). The top 25% of scores formed the second peak in the distribution and is designated to the right of the dotted line in the figure. For each skeletal malocclusion subsequently discussed, emphasis is placed on the higher tier of studies and the effect that orthognathic surgery had on TMD signs and symptoms.

MANDIBULAR RETROGNATHISM: EFFECTS OF ORTHOGNATHIC SURGERY ON INCIDENTAL TEMPOROMANDIBULAR DISORDER SIGNS AND SYMPTOMS

Patients with class II skeletal malocclusions corrected by a BSSO ($\pm$Le Fort I osteotomy) were examined for changes in TMD signs and symptoms in 23 publications (3 publications examined the same data set) (see **Table 1**). Six of these

Table 3
Description and examples of bias in clinical studies

Experimental Bias	Description	Example
Sampling bias	Sample does not reflect the characteristics of the general population under study	Patient sample acquired from referrals to a practice/university or consecutive patients encountered in practice
Selection bias	Sample is not a homogenous group of patients with similar characteristics	Studies that do not have specific inclusion/exclusion criteria may have a nonhomogenous group of patients
Response bias	TMD questionnaires are used to determine previous and current pain levels. Also, the questions may depend on the patient's memory of pain	Questionnaires sent to patients are returned by a motivated or interested subset and the characteristics of these patients may not represent the general population Memory of pain has been shown not to be accurate
Measurement bias	Data acquisition lacks reliable and valid measurement techniques and this can bias the measures	Examiners are not calibrated regarding assessment of TMD variables such as TMJ and muscle pain, joint sounds, and mandibular range of motion
Procedural bias	Interaction and time spent with the patient is not standardized and may bias the study	Lack of a scripted set of questions during the clinical interview
Outcome reporting bias	Data are selectively omitted before statistical analysis and these are reported in the publication	No studies in the review of literature examined this issue. However, approximately 66% of clinical neurology publications had such major discrepancies

Table 4
Research design criteria for assessment of clinical studies

Study Design	Points
Type of Study	
Retrospective	1
Prospective	3
Randomized, prospective	5
Control Group	
None	0
Unmatched	2
Age and sex matched	5
Calibrated/Blinded Examiners	
None	0
Calibrated or blinded	3
Calibrated and blinded	5
Well-defined Inclusion/Exclusion Criteria	
None	0
Inclusion or exclusion criteria	2
Both inclusion and exclusion criteria	4
Well-defined Skeletal Malocclusion Group	
Not reported	0
Mix of skeletal malocclusion groups	1
Single skeletal malocclusion groups assessed	5
Well-defined Orthognathic Surgery Type	
Not reported	0
Mix of maxillary/mandibular surgeries	1
Single maxillary or mandibular surgery assessed	5
TMD Assessment	
Questionnaire	1
Clinical signs/symptoms (variable)	2
Modified validated criteria (ie, modified Helkimo index)	4
Validated criteria (RDC for TMD, CMI, Helkimo index)	6
Follow-up Duration	
Not reported	0
6 mo or less	2
1 y	4
2 y or greater	6
Statistics	
None	0
Descriptive statistics	2
Inferential: univariate	4
Inferential: multivariate	6

publications were found to be in the top 25% of the studies reviewed.[26,28,33,37,41,43] After review of the top publications, the impact of orthognathic surgery on TMD signs and symptoms in this group of patients was mixed at a 2-year follow-up assessment. In 1 study, a counterclockwise rotation of the mandible with at least a 7-mm advancement caused an increase in muscle and TMJ pain, whereas a clockwise rotation had no effect.[41] In 3 other studies, there was no statistical difference between preoperative and postoperative assessments.[28,33,43] This lack of statistical difference can be attributed to the small number of patients that participated in the studies, resulting in an underpowered ability to detect statistical differences. In addition, in 2 studies, overall muscle pain[26] or TMJ pain[37] was reduced on postsurgical assessment at 2 years. However, in 1 study, approximately 25% of patients had an increase in the muscle index score, demonstrating the variability in the response to orthognathic surgery (see Figure 1 in Rodrigues-Garcia and colleagues[26]). Based on the current literature, a mandibular advancement greater than 7 mm combined with a counterclockwise rotation seems to increase the risk of postoperative masticatory muscle and TMJ pain, whereas smaller advancements with a counterclockwise rotation have a predominant effect on increasing muscle symptoms.

MANDIBULAR PROGNATHISM: EFFECTS OF ORTHOGNATHIC SURGERY ON INCIDENTAL TEMPOROMANDIBULAR DISORDER SIGNS AND SYMPTOMS

Twenty-two publications were identified describing correction of class III skeletal malocclusions and

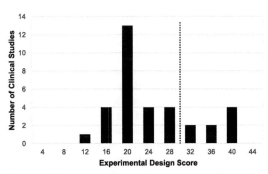

Fig. 1. Histogram of assessment scores for rating research design biases in clinical studies of orthognathic surgery and TMD. The vertical dotted line divides the top 25% of studies (*right side* of *dotted line*) from the lower 75% of studies (*left side* of *dotted line*). These top 25% represent the best of the reviewed studies that were found in the current literature.

evaluating TMD signs and symptoms (see **Table 1**). Of these publications, 4 were in the top 25% of all studies reviewed.[10,33,37,43] Two of the 4 publications found no overall difference in TMD signs and symptoms between preoperative and postoperative assessments at 1-year[39] and 2-year[33] follow-ups. Again, the lack of statistical difference could be caused by the small number of patients examined in each study. The other 2 studies found a significant decrease in the frequency of masticatory muscle pain[43] and/or TMJ arthralgia[10,43] at 6-month or 3-year follow-up, but individual responses varied.[10] However, in contrast with class II skeletal malocclusion correction, there was a consistent overall reduction in TMD signs and symptoms.

APERTOGNATHIA: EFFECTS OF ORTHOGNATHIC SURGERY ON INCIDENTAL TEMPOROMANDIBULAR DISORDER SIGNS AND SYMPTOMS

Although 9 studies were identified in the literature review, none of the studies that evaluated only apertognathia were in the top 25% of studies. Most of the studies addressed anterior open-bite presentation in combination with correction of another skeletal malocclusion. Therefore, it was not possible to isolate the effects of correcting apertognathia on TMD signs and symptoms.

PRIMARY PATIENTS WITH TEMPOROMANDIBULAR DISORDER: EFFECTS OF ORTHOGNATHIC SURGERY ON SIGNS AND SYMPTOMS

Only 1 study was identified that compared patients with class III TMD treated using reversible treatment approaches before orthognathic surgery with patients with TMD treated only by orthognathic surgery.[10] This study had a small number of patients per group (n = 15). Self-reported symptoms were evaluated by a questionnaire, whereas clinical signs and symptoms were assessed using the research diagnostic criteria (RDC) for TMD criteria. Using these data, the investigators concluded that treating the TMD signs and symptoms before surgery had no effect on reducing postoperative TMD signs and symptoms compared with orthognathic surgery alone. Both groups of class III patients were reported to have a reduction in signs and symptoms.

DISCUSSION

The concept of primary treatment of TMDs using orthognathic surgery is not consistent with the current evidence-based approach to using reversible therapies. However, knowledge of the impact of orthognathic surgery on preexisting TMD conditions, or of their causing masticatory muscle or TMJ pain and dysfunction when none is present before surgery, is important for appropriate surgical planning and postsurgical management. Although there is a need for additional, well-controlled studies to refine knowledge on this topic, there are a few studies that have provided insight into potential TMD complications after class II and class III skeletal malocclusion correction. In studies that have minimized investigation bias, class III correction seems to have an overall minimal effect on the masticatory muscles and TMJs in the follow-up time frame of 2 to 3 years. Class II correction seems to reduce the overall frequency of TMD signs and symptoms with the exception of those cases that require greater than 7 mm of mandibular advancement and a counterclockwise rotation of the mandible or only a counterclockwise rotation. The type of mandibular fixation (ie, rigid or nonrigid fixation) also has not been shown to elicit or increase TMD signs and symptoms after orthognathic surgery.

Studies of patients with preexisting TMD conditions that were treated using orthognathic surgery are limited in number. However, based on the study outcomes for TMD in patients with class III malocclusion treated by a BSSO and Le Fort I osteotomy, the frequency of TMD signs and symptoms was not increased and, when present, both TMJ pain and noise were significantly reduced. However, individual responses varied. The lack of studies of other skeletal deformities, and the effect of orthognathic surgery on preexisting TMDs, limits interpretation of orthognathic surgery procedures as reliable techniques to reduce or eliminate TMD signs and symptoms.

This article clearly shows that most studies use orthodontic treatment before surgery and after surgery to refine the occlusion. However, these studies have not addressed the impact of orthodontics on TMD signs and symptoms. Most of the studies were underpowered statistically to determine this impact. Incorporation of an orthodontic control group that is age and sex matched and has the same timing of TMD assessment as the orthodontic/surgical treatment group might identify the possibility of the interaction of orthodontic treatment and orthognathic surgery on TMDs. The number of patients that would be required in each group to achieve sufficient statistical power to detect differences in TMD outcomes between experimental and control groups seems to be greater than 125 based on the work of Frey and colleagues.[41]

This article also emphasizes the need to minimize investigational biases observed in clinical studies that have included orthognathic surgery/TMD outcomes assessment. In our evaluation of the literature, assessment criteria for rating clinical studies were compiled and used to provide a means of comparing each clinical study that was reviewed. Most of the studies did not adequately address various biases that are encountered in clinical research. Thus, there is a need for additional well-designed studies to continue to explore the potential impact of orthognathic surgery on TMD signs and symptoms.

SUMMARY

The currently available evidence in the literature does not support most orthognathic surgical interventions for correction of class II malocclusions, class III malocclusions, or apertognathia as a cause of postoperative temporomandibular disorders. The exception seems to be a counterclockwise rotation of the mandible after a BSSO procedure, which has been shown to be associated with an increase in masticatory muscle pain. When this counterclockwise rotation is combined with a mandibular advancement of greater than 7 mm, both masticatory myalgia and TMJ arthralgia were found to increase in prevalence. Patients who have a preexisting TMD and have a class III skeletal malocclusion may experience an overall reduction in the frequency of TMJ pain and noise. However, individual responses are variable and some patients have an increase in TMD signs and symptoms. Therefore, more studies incorporating appropriate sex-matched and age-matched controls, controls for the effects of orthodontics before orthognathic surgery, and adequate sample sizes to allow for adequate statistical power to test for differences between patient and control groups are required to confirm these earlier results.

REFERENCES

1. Ta LE, Dionne RA. Treatment of painful temporomandibular joints with a cyclooxygenase-2 inhibitor: a randomized placebo-controlled comparison of celecoxib to naproxen. Pain 2004; 111(1–2):13–21.
2. Haggman-Henrikson B, Alstergren P, Davidson T, et al. Pharmacological treatment of orofacial pain - health technology assessment including a systematic review with network meta-analysis. J Oral Rehabil 2017;44(10):800–26.
3. Herman CR, Schiffman EL, Look JO, et al. The effectiveness of adding pharmacologic treatment with clonazepam or cyclobenzaprine to patient education and self-care for the treatment of jaw pain upon awakening: a randomized clinical trial. J Orofac Pain 2002;16(1):64–70.
4. Armijo-Olivo S, Pitance L, Singh V, et al. Effectiveness of manual therapy and therapeutic exercise for temporomandibular disorders: systematic review and meta-analysis. Phys Ther 2016;96(1):9–25.
5. Dworkin SF, Huggins KH, Wilson L, et al. A randomized clinical trial using research diagnostic criteria for temporomandibular disorders-axis II to target clinic cases for a tailored self-care TMD treatment program. J Orofac Pain 2002;16(1):48–63.
6. Dworkin SF, Turner JA, Mancl L, et al. A randomized clinical trial of a tailored comprehensive care treatment program for temporomandibular disorders. J Orofac Pain 2002;16(4):259–76.
7. Dao TTT, Lavigne GJ, Charbonneau A, et al. The efficacy of oral splints in the treatment of myofascial pain of the jaw muscles: a controlled clinical trial. Pain 1994;56:85–94.
8. Truelove E, Huggins KH, Mancl L, et al. The efficacy of traditional, low-cost and nonsplint therapies for temporomandibular disorder: a randomized controlled trial. J Am Dent Assoc 2006;137(8): 1099–107 [quiz: 1169].
9. Greene CS, Obrez A. Treating temporomandibular disorders with permanent mandibular repositioning: is it medically necessary? Oral Surg Oral Med Oral Pathol Oral Radiol 2015;119(5):489–98.
10. Yoon SY, Song JM, Kim YD, et al, Pusan Korea Pusan National University. Clinical changes of TMD and condyle stability after two jaw surgery with and without preceding TMD treatments in class III patients. Maxillofac Plast Reconstr Surg 2015;37(1):9.
11. Greene CS. The fallacies of clinical success in dentistry. Joral Med 1976;31:52–5.
12. Greene CS, Mohl ND, McNeill C, et al. Temporomandibular disorders and science: a response to the critics. Am J Orthod Dentofac Orthop 1999;116(4):430–1.
13. Sebastiani AM, Baratto-Filho F, Bonotto D, et al. Influence of orthognathic surgery for symptoms of temporomandibular dysfunction. Oral Surg Oral Med Oral Pathol Oral Radiol 2016;121(2):119–25.
14. Al-Riyami S, Cunningham SJ, Moles DR. Orthognathic treatment and temporomandibular disorders: a systematic review. Part 2. Signs and symptoms and meta-analyses. Am J Orthod dentofacial orthopedics 2009;136(5):626.e1-6 [discussion: 626-627].
15. Al-Moraissi EA, Wolford LM, Perez D, et al. Does orthognathic surgery cause or cure temporomandibular disorders? A systematic review and meta-analysis. J Oral Maxillofac Surg 2017;75(9):1835–47.
16. Upton LG, Scott RF, Hayward JR. Major maxillomandibular malrelations and temporomandibular joint pain-dysfunction. J Prosthet Dent 1984;51:686–90.
17. Karabouta I, Martis C. The TMJ dysfunction syndrome before and after sagittal split osteotomy of the rami. J Maxillofac Surg 1985;13(4):185–8.

18. Timmis DP, Aragon SB, Van Sickels JE. Masticatory dysfunction with rigid and nonrigid osteosynthesis of sagittal split osteotomies. Oral Surg Oral Med Oral Pathol 1986;62(2):119–23.

19. Magnusson T, Ahlborg G, Finne K, et al. Changes in temporomandibular joint pain-dysfunction after surgical correction of dentofacial anomalies. Int J Oral Maxillofac Surg 1986;15(6):707–14.

20. Kerstens HC, Tuinzing DB, van der Kwast WA. Temporomandibular joint symptoms in orthognathic surgery. J Craniomaxillofac Surg 1989; 17(5):215–8.

21. Smith V, Williams B, Stapleford R. Rigid internal fixation and the effects on the temporomandibular joint and masticatory system: a prospective study. Am J Orthod dentofacial orthopedics 1992;102(6):491–500.

22. Athanasiou AE, Melsen B. Craniomandibular dysfunction following surgical correction of mandibular prognathism. Angle Orthod 1992;62(1):9–14.

23. De Clercq CA, Abeloos JS, Mommaerts MY, et al. Temporomandibular joint symptoms in an orthognathic surgery population. J Craniomaxillofac Surg 1995;23(3):195–9.

24. Feinerman DM, Piecuch JF. Long-term effects of orthognathic surgery on the temporomandibular joint: comparison of rigid and nonrigid fixation methods. Int J Oral Maxill Surg 1995;24(4):268–72.

25. Onizawa K, Schmelzeisen R, Vogt S. Alteration of temporomandibular joint symptoms after orthognathic surgery: comparison with healthy volunteers. J Oral Maxillofac Surg 1995;53(2):117–21 [discussion: 122–3].

26. Rodrigues-Garcia RC, Sakai S, Rugh JD, et al. Effects of major class II occlusal corrections on temporomandibular signs and symptoms. J Orofac Pain 1998;12(3):185–92.

27. Panula K, Somppi M, Finne K, et al. Effects of orthognathic surgery on temporomandibular joint dysfunction. A controlled prospective 4-year follow-up study. Int J Oral Maxill Surg 2000;29(3):183–7.

28. Nemeth DZ, Rodrigues-Garcia RC, Sakai S, et al. Bilateral sagittal split osteotomy and temporomandibular disorders: rigid fixation versus wire fixation. Oral Surg Oral Med Oral Pathol Oral Radiol Endod 2000;89(1):29–34.

29. Egermark I, Blomqvist JE, Cromvik U, et al. Temporomandibular dysfunction in patients treated with orthodontics in combination with orthognathic surgery. Eur J Orthod 2000;22(5):537–44.

30. Kobayashi T, Honma K, Hamamoto Y, et al. Effects of wire and miniplate fixation on mandibular stability and TMJ symptoms following orthognathic surgery. Clin Orthod Res 2000;3:155–61.

31. Westermark A, Shayeghi F, Thor A. Temporomandibular dysfunction in 1,516 patients before and after orthognathic surgery. Int J Adult Orthodon Orthognath Surg 2001;16(2):145–51.

32. Aghabeigi B, Hiranaka D, Keith DA, et al. Effect of orthognathic surgery on the temporomandibular joint in patients with anterior open bite. Int J Adult Orthodon Orthognath Surg 2001;16(2):153–60.

33. Dervis E, Tuncer E. Long-term evaluations of temporomandibular disorders in patients undergoing orthognathic surgery compared with a control group. Oral Surg Oral Med Oral Pathol Oral Radiol Endod 2002;94(5):554–60.

34. Ueki K, Marukawa K, Nakagawa K, et al. Condylar and temporomandibular joint disc positions after mandibular osteotomy for prognathism. J Oral Maxillofac Surg 2002;60(12):1424–32 [discussion 1432–4].

35. Wolford LM, Reiche-Fischel O, Mehra P. Changes in temporomandibular joint dysfunction after orthognathic surgery. J Oral Maxillofac Surg 2003;61(6): 655–60 [discussion: 661].

36. Pahkala R, Heino J. Effects of sagittal split ramus osteotomy on temporomandibular disorders in seventy-two patients. Acta Odontol Scand 2004; 62(4):238–44.

37. Borstlap WA, Stoelinga PJ, Hoppenreijs TJ, et al. Stabilisation of sagittal split advancement osteotomies with miniplates: a prospective, multicentre study with two-year follow-up. Part I. Clinical parameters. Int J Oral Maxill Surg 2004;33(5):433–41.

38. Kallela I, Laine P, Suuronen R, et al. Assessment of material- and technique-related complications following sagittal split osteotomies stabilized by biodegradable polylactide screws. Oral Surg Oral Med Oral Pathol Oral Radiol Endod 2005;99(1):4–10.

39. Farella M, Michelotti A, Bocchino T, et al. Effects of orthognathic surgery for class III malocclusion on signs and symptoms of temporomandibular disorders and on pressure pain thresholds of the jaw muscles. Int J Oral Maxill Surg 2007;36(7):583–7.

40. Valle-Corotti K, Pinzan A, do Valle CV, et al. Assessment of temporomandibular disorder and occlusion in treated class III malocclusion patients. J Appl Oral Sci 2007;15(2):110–4.

41. Frey DR, Hatch JP, Van Sickels JE, et al. Effects of surgical mandibular advancement and rotation on signs and symptoms of temporomandibular disorder: a 2-year follow-up study. Am J Orthod Dentofacial Orthop 2008;133(4):490.e1-8.

42. Dujoncquoy JP, Ferri J, Raoul G, et al. Temporomandibular joint dysfunction and orthognathic surgery: a retrospective study. Head Face Med 2010;6:27.

43. Abrahamsson C, Henrikson T, Nilner M, et al. TMD before and after correction of dentofacial deformities by orthodontic and orthognathic treatment. Int J Oral Maxill Surg 2013;42(6):752–8.

44. Togashi M, Kobayashi H, Hasebe D, et al. Effects of surgical orthodontic treatment for dentofacial deformities on signs and symptoms of temporomandibular joint. J Oral Maxillofac Surg Med Pathol 2013; 25:18–23.

45. Mladenovic I, Jovic N, Cutovic T, et al. Temporomandibular disorders after orthognathic surgery in patients with mandibular prognathism with depression as a risk factor. Acta Odontol Scand 2013; 71(1):57–64.

46. Scolozzi P, Wandeler PA, Courvoisier DS. Can clinical factors predict postoperative temporomandibular disorders in orthognathic patients? A retrospective study of 219 patients. Oral Surg Oral Med Oral Pathol Oral Radiol 2015;119(5):531–8.

47. di Paolo C, Pompa G, Arangio P, et al. Evaluation of temporomandibular disorders before and after orthognathic surgery: therapeutic considerations on a sample of 76 patients. J Int Soc Prev Community Dent 2017;7(2):125–9.

48. Kam-Hansen S, Jakubowski M, Kelley JM, et al. Altered placebo and drug labeling changes the outcome of episodic migraine attacks. Sci Transl Med 2014;6(218):218ra215.

49. Scott BA, Clark GM, Hatch JP, et al. Comparing prospective and retrospective evaluations of temporomandibular disorders after orthognathic surgery. J Am Dental Assoc 1997;128(7):999–1003.

50. De Boever AL, Keeling SD, Hilsenbeck S, et al. Signs of temporomandibular disorders in patients with horizontal mandibular deficiency. J Orofac Pain 1996;10(1):21–7.

51. Howard B, Scott JT, Blubaugh M, et al. Systematic review: outcome reporting bias is a problem in high impact factor neurology journals. PLoS One 2017;12(7):e0180986.

Arthroscopy Versus Arthrocentesis for Treating Internal Derangements of the Temporomandibular Joint

Daniel M. Laskin, DDS, MS

KEYWORDS

- Internal derangement • Arthroscopy • Arthrocentesis • Disc displacement • Complications

KEY POINTS

- In treating internal derangements of the temporomandibular joint, re-establishing joint mobility is more important than restoring disc position.
- It is not necessary to visualize the joint to successfully treat internal derangements.
- Arthrocentesis is as effective as arthroscopy in treating internal derangements.
- Arthrocentesis has fewer and less serious complications.

Prior to the early 1970s, the surgical treatment of internal derangements of the temporomandibular joint (TMJ) involved either restoration of the intra-articular disc to its normal position (discoplasty) or removal of the disc (discectomy). However, the introduction of arthroscopic surgery for the management of internal derangements by Ohnishi in 1975[1] and the subsequent development of the technique by Murakami and Ito[2] in Japan and Sanders in the United States[3] represented a major advancement in the treatment of such conditions, because it involved a less invasive approach. Although initially this procedure consisted mainly of irrigation of the joint and the breaking up of adhesions (lysis and lavage), various surgical manipulations similar those performed arthroscopically in other joints were subsequently introduced by some surgeons. It soon became evident that in the treatment of patients with internal derangements, restoring joint mobility rather than disc position was the important factor. This produced a better distribution of forces within the joint, allowed more physiologic function by improving the diffusion of nutriments and the elimination of inflammatory breakdown products, and ultimately resulted in transformation of the painful anteriorly displaced retrodiscal tissue into a more fibrotic functional pseudodisc.[4]

The success reported with arthroscopic management of internal derangements ultimately led to the introduction of arthrocentesis for the treatment of closed lock in the TMJ by Nitzen, Dolwick and Martinez in 1991.[5] This procedure involved lavage of the TMJ via 2 hypodermic needles introduced into the upper joint space and lysis of adhesions hydraulically and by manual manipulation of the mandible. Subsequently, the procedure was also reported to have been used successfully for the treatment of painful TMJ clicking[6] and TMJ osteoarthritis[7] and rheumatoid arthritis.[8]

However, because arthrocentesis does not involve visualization of the joint structures or the use of additional surgical manipulations, it raises the question of whether arthroscopy should be the preferred initial treatment for internal derangements of the TMJ. Because reports on other

Disclosure: The author has nothing to disclose.
Department of Oral and Maxillofacial Surgery, Virginia Commonwealth University School of Dentistry, 521 North 11th Street, Richmond, VA 23298-0566, USA
E-mail address: dmlaskin@vcu.edu

conditions for which arthroscopic surgery and arthrocentesis have been used are limited, this discussion will focus only on internal derangements, comparing both individual studies and those in which both procedures were used by the same surgeons. Because some arthroscopic studies involved only lysis and lavage and others involved lysis and lavage plus such procedures as joint debridement, abrasion arthroplasty, lateral capsular release, lateral pterygoid muscle detachment, and disc repositioning, these 2 groups will also be compared.

ARTHROSCOPY VERSUS ARTHROCENTESIS IN SEPARATE STUDIES

There have been numerous studies in which internal derangements have been treated either arthroscopically or by arthrocentesis. An extensive review of arthroscopic surgery was reported by Israel in 1999,[9] which involved data from 11 studies published between 1987 and 1996. Although most of the 3955 patients had nonreducing anterior disc displacement, some had only clicking. Arthroscopic lysis with lavage was the most frequent procedure, but some patients were also treated with various surgical manipulations. The results showed a mean success rate of 84%, with an average increase in maximum mouth opening of 10.4 mm and 82% of patients reporting less pain. Similar results have been reported by Alvarez and colleagues[10] (61 patients, 4-year follow-up, 81.4% success), Murakami and colleagues[11] (33 patients, 10-year follow-up, 83.8% success), Sorel and Piecuch[12] (22 patients, 2 to 10.8-year follow-up, 91% success), and White[13] (66 patients, 8-year follow-up, 76% success). The average success rate for these 5 studies is 83%.

The long-term effectiveness of arthrocentesis was reported to be 85% by Frost and colleagues[14] (40 patients, 14-month follow-up). Nitzen, Samson, and Better[15] reported a 95% success rate, whereas Hosaka and colleagues[16] reported 79% success (20 patients, 3-year follow-up), and Carvajal and Laskin[17] had an 88% success rate (26 patients, 49 months). The mean success rate for these 4 studies is 87%. In a review of 14 articles from the international literature, Al-Belasy and Dolwick[18] found an 83.2% success rate. Thus, based on individual studies, arthrocentesis is as effective as arthroscopy for the treatment of internal derangements.

ARTHROSCOPY VERSUS ARTHROCENTESIS IN THE SAME STUDIES

Because of the possible variations in individual studies, as well as the greater potential for bias,

they are not as reliable as comparative studies done at a single institution. A review of the literature revealed 2 such early studies[19,20] that should arthroscopy to be somewhat better, but since that time 5 studies[21–25] in which this type of comparison was made, showed no significant difference (**Table 1**).

DISCUSSION

The results of the preceding comparisons provide strong evidence that the 2 procedures are comparable in effectiveness. However, it has been claimed that arthroscopic surgery has the advantage of allowing the surgeon to look into the joint and directly treat any pathology that exists. To address this issue, one needs to compare the results from studies on arthroscopic lysis and lavage alone with studies on lysis and lavage plus other surgical maneuvers reported in the literature. **Table 2** shows that there is no significant difference. Moreover, in 2 comparison studies of arthroscopic lysis and lavage with lysis and lavage plus arthroscopic surgery from the same institution by Gonzalez-Garcia and colleagues,[31,32] no statistical difference was noted. Thus, if lysis with lavage alone is effective, it is not necessary to look into the joint, and arthrocentesis can be the initial treatment for internal derangements.

Other advantages of arthrocentesis include less invasiveness, no need for special instruments, less postoperative morbidity, lower cost, and low potential for complications. The numerous complications of arthroscopic surgery are listed in **Box 1**.[33] The only significant complication of arthrocentesis has been 1 case of an extradural hematoma.[34]

The successful management of patients with close lock using arthrocentesis, despite the fact that the intra-articular disc is still in an anteriorly

Table 1	
Success of arthroscopy and arthrocentesis compared in the same study	
Author	**Arthroscopy Arthrocentesis**
Kropmans et al,[21] 1999	No significant difference
Goudot et al,[22] 2000	No significant difference
Sanroman.[23] 2004	No significant difference
Hobeich et al,[24] 2007	No significant difference
Tan & Krishnaswamy,[25] 2012	No significant difference

Table 2
Success treating temporomandibular joint internal derangements with arthroscopic lysis and lavage alone or with arthroscopic surgery added

Lysis and Lavage		Lysis, Lavage +Surgery	
Sanders & Buoncristiani,[26] 1987	90%	Moses & Poker,[28] 1989	92%
Indresano,[27] 1989	83%	Davis et al,[29] 1991	86%
Sorel & Piecuch,[12] 2000	91%	Mosby,[30] 1993	93%
Fridrich et al,[19] 1996	82%		*90%*
Murakami et al,[20] 1995	91%		
		87.4%	

displaced position, indicates that the ultimate key to success involves the improved joint movement rather than the temporary removal of cytokines and inflammatory tissue breakdown products. Thus, not only is hydraulic lysis of adhesions important, but also active manual manipulation of the joint during the procedure. It has been shown that this is best accomplished with the patient under general anesthesia rather than when subjected to local anesthesia plus sedation.[35] Another factor in the long-term success of TMJ arthrocentesis for internal derangements is management of the cause of the problem as well as the symptoms. This means that postoperatively those patients in whom chronic parafunction is the contributing factor must wear a bite appliance at night to prevent clenching and grinding.

Box 1
Reported complications with temporomandibular joint arthroscopy

- Arteriovenous fistula
- Pseudoaneurysm
- Facial, trigeminal, auditory nerve injury
- Infection (otitis media, TMJ, infratemporal fossa)
- Broken instruments in the joint
- Lateral pharyngeal extravasation
- Extradural hematoma
- Perforation of tympanic membrane and deafness

SUMMARY

The similarity of success in treating internal derangements of the temporomandibular joint with arthroscopy or arthrocentesis, plus the advantage of greater simplicity, lower cost, and fewer complications of the latter procedure, suggests that it should generally be the initial treatment in most instances. Although there have been a few studies on the successful use of arthrocentesis for osteoarthritis and rheumatoid arthritis, further investigation of its effectiveness and comparison to arthroscopic management are needed.

REFERENCES

1. Ohnishi M. Arthroscopy of the temporomandibular joint. J Stomatol Soc Japan 1975;42:207–12.
2. Murakami K, Ito K. Arthroscopy of the temporomandibular joint. In: Watanabe M, editor. Arthroscopy of small joints. Tokyo: Igaku Shoin; 1985. p. 128–39.
3. Sanders B. Arthroscopic surgery of the temporomandibular joint: treatment of internal derangement with persistent closed lock. Oral Surg Oral Med Oral Pathol 1986;62:361–4.
4. Laskin DM. Internal derangements. In: Laskin DM, Greene CS, Hylander W, editors. Temporomandibular disorders: an evidenced-based approach to diagnosis and treatment. Chicago: Quintessence Publishing Co; 2006. p. 249–53.
5. Nitzen DW, Dolwick MF, Martinez GA. Temporomandibular joint arthrocentesis: a simplified treatment for severe, limited mouth opening. J Oral Maxillofac Surg 1991;49:1163–7.
6. Yoda T, Imai H, Shinjyo Y, et al. Effect of arthrocentesis on TMJ disturbance of mouth closure with loud clicking: a preliminary study. Cranio 2002;20:18–22.
7. Nitzen DW, Svidovsky J, Zini A, et al. Effect of arthrocentesis on symptomatic osteoarthritis of the temporomandibular joint and analysis of the effect of preoperative clinical and radiologic features. J Oral Maxillofac Surg 2017;75:260–7.
8. Trieger M, Huffman CH, Rodrigues E. The effect of arthrocentesis of the temporomandibular joint in patients with rheumatoid arthritis. J Oral Maxillofac Surg 1999;57:537–40.
9. Israel HA. The use of arthroscopic surgery for the treatment of temporomandibular disorders. J Oral Maxillofac Surg 1999;57:579–82.
10. Alvarez J, Barbier L, Carmelo Marin J, et al. Temporomandibular arthroscopy: a retrospective clinical study (1995-1999) of 61 cases. Med Oral 2001;6:383–90.
11. Murakami KL, Segami N, Okamoto M, et al. Outcome of arthroscopic surgery for internal

derangements of the temporomandibular joint: long-term results covering 10 years. J Craniomaxillofac Surg 2000;28:264–71.

12. Sorel B, Piecuch JF. Long-term evaluation following emporomandibular joint arathroscopy wih lysis and lavage. J Oral Maxillofac Surg 2000;29:259–63.

13. White RD. Arthroscopic lysis and lavage for internal derangements of the temporomandibular joint. J Oral Maxillofac Surg 2001;59:313–6.

14. Frost DE, Kendell BD, Owsley T. Clinical results in 40 cases. Br J Oral Maxillofac Surg 1992;30:285.

15. Nitzen DW, Samson B, Better H. Long-term outcome of arthrocentesis for severe closed lock of the temporomandibular joint. J Oral Maxillofac Surg 1997;55:151–8.

16. Hosaka H, Murakami K, Goto K, et al. Outcome of arthrocentesis for temporomandibular joint with closed lock at 3 year follow-up. Oral Surg Oral Med Oral Pathol 1996;82:501–4.

17. Carvajal WA, Laskin DM. Long-term evaluation of arthrocentesis for the treatment of internal derangements of the temporomandibular joint. J Oral Maxillofac Surg 2000;58:852–5.

18. Al-Belasy FA, Dolwick MF. Arthrocentesis for the treatment of temporomandibular joint closed lock: a review article. Int J Oral Maxillofac Surg 2007;36: 773–82.

19. Fridrich KL, Wise JM, Zeitler DL. Prospective comparison of arthroscopy and arthrocentesis for temporomandibular joint disorders. J Oral Maxillofac Surg 1996;54:816–20.

20. Murakami K, Hosaka H, Moriya Y, et al. Short-term outcome study for the management of temporomandibular joint closed lock: a comparison of arthrocentesis to nonsurgery and arthroscopic lysis and lavage. Oral Surg Oral Med Oral Pathol 1995;80: 253–7.

21. Kropmans TJ, Dijjstra PU, Stegenga B, et al. Therapeutic outcome assessment in permanent temporomandibular joint disc displacement. J Oral Rehabil 1999;26:357–63.

22. Goudot P, Jaquinet AR, Hugonnet S, et al. Improvement of pain and function after arthroscopy and arthrocentesis of the temporomandibular joint: a comparative study. J Craniomaxillofac Surg 2000; 28:39–43.

23. Sanroman JF. Closed lock (MRI fixed disc): a comparison of arthrocentesis and arthroscopy. Int J Oral Maxillofac Surg 2004;33:344–8.

24. Hobeich JB, Salameh ZA, Ismail E, et al. Arthroscopy versus arthrocentesis. A retrospective study of disc displacement without reduction management. Saudi Med J 2007;28:1541–4.

25. Tan DBP, Krishnaswamy G. A retrospective study of temporomandibular joint internal derangement treated with arthrocentesis and arthroscopy. Proc Singap Healthc 2012;21:73–8.

26. Sanders B, Buoncristiani R. Diagnostic and surgical arthroscopy of the temporomandibular joint: clinical experience with 137 procedures over a 2-year period. J Craniomandib Disord 1987;1:202–13.

27. Indresano AT. Arthroscopic surgery of the temporomandibular joint: report of 64 patients with long-term follow-up. J Oral Maxillofac Surg 1989; 47:439–41.

28. Moses JJ, Poker ID. TMJ arthroscopic surgery: an analysis of 237 patients. J Oral Maxillofac Surg 1989;47:439–41.

29. Davis EL, Kaminishi RM, Marshall MW. Arthroscopic surgery for treatment of closed lock. J Oral Maxillofac Surg 1991;49:704–7.

30. Mosby EL. Efficacy of temporomandibular joint arthroscopy: a retrospective study. J Oral Maxillofac Surg 1993;51:17–21.

31. Gonzalez-Garcia R, Rodriguez-Campo FJ, Monje F, et al. Operative versus simple arthroscopic surgery for chronic closed lock of the temporomandibular joint: a clinical study of 344 arthroscopic procedures. Int J Oral Maxillofac Surg 2008;37: 790–6.

32. Gonzalez-Garcia R, Rodriguez-Campo FJ. Arthroscopic lysis and lavage versus operative arthroscopy in the outcome of temporomandibular joint internal derangement: a comparative study based on Wilkes stages. J Oral Maxillofac Surg 2011;69: 2513–24.

33. Masashi T, Toshirou K, Seto K, et al. Complications of temporomandibular joint arthroscopy: a retrospective analysis of 301 lysis and lavage procedures performed usin the triangulation technique. J Oral Maxillofac Surg 2000;58:500–5.

34. Carroll TA, Smith K, Jakubowski J. Extradural haematoma following temporomandibular joint arthrocentesis and lavage. Br J Neurosurg 2000;14:152–4.

35. Mehra P, Arya V. TMJ arthrocentesis: outcomes under intravenous sedation vs general anesthesia. J Oral Maxillofac Surg 2015;73:834–42.

Discectomy Versus Disc Preservation for Internal Derangement of the Temporomandibular Joint

Shravan Kumar Renapurkar, BDS, DMD

KEYWORDS

- Internal derangement • Discectomy • Discopexy • Discoplasty

KEY POINTS

- Arthrocentesis or arthroscopic surgery should be the initial treatment in patients with internal derangement who do not respond to nonsurgical therapy.
- Arthrotomy should be reserved for patients who fail minimally invasive procedures.
- Discs with good form and mobility, and with minimal or no perforation, should be preserved to keep the joint structure intact.
- Nonsalvageable, dysfunctional discs with large perforations and a lack of mobility require discectomy.
- None of the alloplastic or autogenous disc replacements have proven superior to discectomy alone.

The term internal derangement of the temporomandibular joint (TMJ) relates to an abnormal relationship between the articular disc, the condyle, and the eminence that interferes with proper joint function. The terms disc derangement and disc displacement are often used interchangeably with internal derangement.[1,2] Although the 12-o-clock position for the posterior band of the disc is considered normal, an even more anteriorly positioned disc has been suggested to be a variation of normal in many studies of asymptomatic subjects.[3–5]

In recent years, medical management and minimally invasive treatment of internal derangements have decreased the frequency of arthrotomy-based procedures.[4] The success of minimally invasive procedures, such as arthroscopy and arthrocentesis, which do not significantly affect the disc position, provides further evidence that its precise location may not be critical in the pathogenesis and treatment of internal derangements (See Daniel M Laskin's article, "Arthroscopy Versus Arthrocentesis for Treating Internal Derangements of the Temporomandibular Joint," in this issue). Nevertheless, TMJ discopexy/discoplasty and discectomy still play an important role in management for symptomatic, dysfunctional patients with internal derangements that do not respond to less invasive treatment.

CLINICAL DIAGNOSIS AND CLASSIFICATION OF INTERNAL DERANGEMENTS

Diagnosis of disc displacement with or without reduction is based on a combination of the history, clinical examination, and findings on an MRI, which shows the position and shape of the disc in the open and closed mouth position, joint

Disclosure: The author has nothing to disclose.
Department of Oral and Maxillofacial Surgery, Virginia Commonwealth University, 520 North 12th Street, Wood Building, Room 311C, Richmond, VA 23298, USA
E-mail address: srenapurkar@vcu.edu

Oral Maxillofacial Surg Clin N Am 30 (2018) 329–333
https://doi.org/10.1016/j.coms.2018.05.002
1042-3699/18/

effusion, and any degenerative changes in the joint. Although the exact cause of internal derangements is unknown, proposed factors include microtrauma or macrotrauma, parafunctional habits, laxity of the joint soft tissues, and changes in the composition of the synovial fluid.[3]

Although clicking is a frequent clinical sign indicating anterior disc displacement with reduction, other causes, such as hypermobility of TMJ or joint pathology, should be ruled out. Asymptomatic clicking is common in 30% to 40% of the population and is not considered an indication for intervention.[2,6] The most commonly used classification of internal derangements is that proposed by Wilkes, which shows the progression of the disease.

CURRENT EVIDENCE FOR DISC PRESERVATION

Discopexy or discoplasty involves an arthrotomy followed by repair/reshaping and/or repositioning of the intra-articular disc. Disc repositioning was first described in 1979 by McCarty and Farrar[7] and, although supported by numerous retrospective case studies since then, is still surrounded by some skepticism. They reported 94% success in 327 patients over a 6-year period, but the criteria for success were not clearly defined. Various other authors also have reported a high success rate (80%–94%) from disc repositioning and repair.[7–17] A retrospective survey-based study with a mean 20-year follow-up (range, 18–22 years) on patients who underwent disc repositioning showed a 94% improvement in quality of life and 77% reduction in pain at rest, with only one patient requiring subsequent surgery that was attributed to a post-traumatic malocclusion.[18] However, long-term studies have shown that even though there is improvement in clinical signs and symptoms the disc position remains the same.[19]

Discopexy has been reported to be effective even when done with arthroscopic methods.[20] However, a meta-analysis comparing arthroscopy with lysis and lavage, arthroscopic surgery, and open joint surgery in patients with an internal derangement showed that open surgery was more effective in pain reduction than arthroscopic surgery, while having similar outcomes in maximal incisal opening and jaw function.[21]

In summary, the literature supports the concept that a disc that is structurally intact, with a healthy appearance and adequate mobility to allow repositioning without tension, should be salvaged.[8,22] Although disc-preservation surgery has been reported to be successful, there is considerable variability among the techniques used by various surgeons, including the addition of eminectomy, partial disc plication, use of Mitek anchors, and concomitant orthognathic surgery.[8,23,24]

CURRENT EVIDENCE FOR DISCECTOMY

Discectomy is often performed when a dysfunctional, deformed disc cannot be salvaged. Several long-term follow-up studies support the efficacy of discectomy in reducing pain and dysfunction.[25–28] Those studies that suggest the use of discectomy as the primary treatment of an internal derangement of the TMJ are based on claims that discopexy ultimately fails and eventually leads to discectomy, but this assumption is not supported by the evidence.[29]

Heterogeneity in patient populations, low numbers of subjects, variability in patient selection, and the retrospective, nonrandomized nature of the studies make reaching conclusions about the efficacy of discectomy difficult. Morphologic changes in the condyles after discectomy in animal and human studies show an association of discectomy with degenerative joint disease.[30,31] Changes reported include condylar flattening, sclerosis of the condylar surface, osteophyte formation, soft tissue thickening in the joint space, and pseudodisc formation.[26,32–34] The initial bony changes in the condyle have been reported to stabilize over time.[32] Some reports have correlated advanced degenerative changes after discectomy to early loading of the joint and have suggested caution with joint loading for the first 6 months postoperatively.[35] However, these changes have also been reported in unoperated joints, in the contralateral TMJ after unilateral discectomy, in cases of discopexy, and when the disc is replaced with autogenous grafts.[28,36] Such findings in joints that did not undergo discectomy question the causal relationship with absence of the disc. Rather, these condylar changes could represent functional adaptive changes rather than degenerative changes.[26]

CHOICE FOR REPLACEMENT OF THE DISC

There are instances when discopexy or discoplasty are not possible and disc removal is necessary. This raises the question of whether disc replacement is necessary. Although the procedure of discectomy without any replacement was first described by Boman in 1947, concern about subsequent advanced degenerative changes in the condyle and persistent symptoms in some patients led surgeons to believe that replacement was necessary.[37,38] This presumed causal role of discectomy in the pathogenesis of TMJ osteoarthritis has resulted in the development of numerous autogenous and alloplastic disc replacement options.

Silicone rubber sheet (Silastic, Dow Corning Corporation, Midland, MI) was initially used as a permanent disc replacement, but it was subsequently abandoned because of poor wear properties and foreign body reactions.[39–41] Use of Silastic as a temporary disc replacement to prevent adhesions in the TMJ and help formation of a capsule that could act as a pseudodisc also has been reported to result in severe condylar lesions.[42,43] Proplast-Teflon (Vitek, Inc, Houston, TX) also was reported to have a high success rate in the short term, but it was eventually shown to cause a foreign body giant cell reaction resulting in severe condylar resorption.[44–46] The Food and Drug Administration subsequently cautioned against the use of silicone rubber and Proplast-Teflon as TMJ implants and the latter was taken off the market in 1988 and a recall of patients with such implants was issued in 1990.[47]

Autogenous TMJ disc replacements have gained popularity because of the problems faced with alloplastic disc replacements. These are biocompatible and easily harvested, although they may require additional extension of the incision (temporalis flap) or an additional surgical site (auricular graft, abdominal dermal-fat grafts).

There are only a few studies evaluating the temporalis myofascial flap as a replacement for the disc, with most reporting its use in cases of ankylosis or in patients with failed previous alloplastic replacements.[48,49] Auricular cartilage grafts, although reported to be successful in many studies, have subsequently shown fibrosis and fragmentation.[50–53] Dimitroulis reported the use of abdominal dermal-fat grafts to have good outcomes in improving joint function, quality of life, and decreasing pain and joint noise, but radiographic review showed that they failed to prevent condylar changes in a significant number of patients, especially in those who had prior condylar surgery.[36,54,55] Moreover, a recent retrospective study comparing discectomy alone and discectomy with an abdominal dermis-fat graft showed no significant difference in symptom improvement.[56]

A recent meta-analysis comparing discectomy without replacement with discectomy with autogenous interpositional grafts showed similar mean success rates for all groups (discectomy alone, 86.5%; temporalis flap, 91.4%; auricular cartilage graft, 82.4%; dermal graft, 87.9%).[57] Based on these findings there seems to be no superiority of interpositional grafts over discectomy alone. Tissue-engineered disc replacement may be the ultimate solution, but this is still in the nascent stages of development without reliable evidence for clinical use.

SUMMARY

Surgical treatment of internal derangements of TMJ should only be considered when nonsurgical options fail. Minimally invasive options, such as arthrocentesis or arthroscopic surgery, although they do not address the position of the disc, are generally efficacious in reducing the pain and dysfunction associated with disc derangement. Arthrotomy-based surgical options, although used less frequently than in the past, still have an important role in managing patients who do not respond to conservative treatment. However, discectomy should not be the primary surgery. Discopexy or discoplasty are the initial surgical treatments of choice. Only discs that are highly deformed, perforated, dysfunctional, and lack mobility should be removed. In such cases, replacement is not indicated because none of the current replacement options have data to show superiority over discectomy alone.

REFERENCES

1. De Leeuw R. Internal derangements of the temporomandibular joint. Oral Maxillofacial Surg Clin North America 2008;20(2):159–68.
2. Larheim TA, Westesson P, Sano T. Temporomandibular joint disk displacement: comparison in asymptomatic volunteers and patients. Radiology 2001;218:428–32.
3. Dijkgraaf LC, de Bont LG, Otten E, et al. Three-dimensional visualization of the temporomandibular joint: a computerized multisectional autopsy study of disc position and configuration. J Oral Maxillofac Surg 1992;50(1):2–10.
4. Stegenga D, Lambert GM. TMJ disc derangements. In: Laskin DM, Greene CS, Hylander WL, editors. TMDs, an evidence-based approach to diagnosis and treatment. Chicago: Quintessence; 2006. p. 441–53.
5. Nitzan DW, Dolwick MF, Martinez GA. Temporomandibular joint arthrocentesis: a simplified treatment for severe, limited mouth opening. J Oral Maxillofac Surg 1991;49:1163.
6. Greene CS, Laskin DM. Long-term status of TMJ clicking in patients with myofascial pain and dysfunction. J Am Dent Assoc 1988;117(3):461–5.

7. McCarty WL, Farrar WB. Surgery for internal derangements of the temporomandibular joint. J Prosthet Dent 1979;42:191.

8. Dolwick MF. Disc preservation surgery for the treatment of internal derangements of the temporomandibular joint. J Oral Maxillofac Surg 2001;59:1047.

9. Mercuri LG, Campbell RL, Shamaskin RG. Intra-articular meniscus dysfunction surgery. A preliminary report. Oral Surg Oral Med Oral Pathol 1982;54:613.

10. Hall MB. Meniscoplasty of the displaced temporomandibular joint meniscus without violating the inferior joint space. J Oral Maxillofac Surg 1984;42:788.

11. Hall MB, Kim M-R, Dolwick MF. Partial thickness plication of the TMJ disc in 149 joints. J Oral Maxillofac Surg 1989;475:140.

12. Dolwick MF, Sanders B. TMJ internal derangement and arthrosis: surgical atlas. St Louis (MO): CV Mosby; 1985.

13. Walker RV, Kalamchi S. A surgical technique for management of internal derangement of the temporomandibular joint. J Oral Maxillofac Surg 1987;45:299.

14. Kerstens HC, Tuinzing DB, van der Kwat WA. Eminectomy and discoplasty for correction of the displaced temporomandibular joint disc. J Oral Maxillofac Surg 1989;47:150.

15. Elias AC, Weber W. Surgical resolution of internal derangements of the temporomandibular joint. J Oral Maxillofac Surg 1990;485:147.

16. Dolwick MF, Nitzan DW. TMJ disk surgery: 8-year follow-up evaluation. Fortschr Kiefer Gesichtschir 1990;35:162.

17. Dolwick MF, Nitzan DW. The role of disc-repositioning surgery for internal derangements of the temporomandibular joint. Oral Maxillofac Surg Clin North Am 1994;6:271.

18. Abramowicz S, Dolwick MF. 20-year follow-up study of disc repositioning surgery for temporomandibular joint internal derangement. J Oral Maxillofacial Surg 2010;68(2):239–42.

19. Montgomery MT, Gordon SM, VanSickels JE, et al. Changes in signs and symptoms following temporomandibular joint disc repositioning surgery. J Oral Maxillofac Surg 1992;50:320.

20. McCain JP, Hossameldin RH, Srouji S, et al. Arthroscopic discopexy is effective in managing temporomandibular joint internal derangement in patients with Wilkes stage II and III. J Oral Maxillofacial Surg 2015;73(3):391–401.

21. Al-Moraissi EA. Open versus arthroscopic surgery for the management of internal derangement of the temporomandibular joint: a meta-analysis of the literature. Int J Oral Maxillofac Surg 2015;44:763–70.

22. Dolwick MF. Intra-articular disc displacement. Part I: Its questionable role in temporomandibular joint pathology. J Oral Maxillofac Surg 1995;53:1069.

23. Silver CML. Long-term results of meniscectomy of the temporomandibular joint. Cranio 1984;3:46–57.

24. Mehra P, Wolford LM. The Mitek mini anchor for TMJ disc repositioning: surgical technique and results. Int J Oral Maxillofac Surg 2001;30(6):497–503.

25. Holmlund AB, Gynther GW, Axelsson S. Diskectomy in treatment of internal derangement of the temporomandibular joint. Follow-up at 1, 3 and 5 years. J Oral Maxillofac Surg 1993;76:972–1071.

26. Eriksson L, Westesson P-L. Long–term evaluation of meniscectomy of the temporomandibular joint. J Oral Maxillofac Surg 1985;43:263–6.

27. Tolvanem M, Oikarinen VJ, Wolf J. A 30 year follow-up study of temporomandibular joint menisctomies: a report of 5 patients. Br J Oral Maxillofac Surg 1988;26:311–3.

28. Takaku S, Toyoda T. Long-term evaluation of diskectomy of the temporomandibular joint. J Oral Maxillofac Surg 1994;52:722–6.

29. Miloro M, Henriksen B. Discectomy as the primary surgical option for internal derangement of the temporomandibular joint. J Oral Maxillofacial Surg 2010;68(4):782–9.

30. Hinton RJ. Alteration in rat condylar cartilage following discectomy. J Dent Res 1992;71:1292.

31. Widmark G, Dahlstrom L, Kahnberg K-E, et al. Diskectomy in the temporomandibular joint with internal derangement: a follow-up study. Oral Surg Oral Med Oral Pathol Oral Radiol Endod 1997;83:314.

32. Agerberg G, Lundberg M. Changes in the temporomandibular joint after surgical treatment. Oral Surg Oral Med Oral Pathol 1971;32:865.

33. Westesson P-L, Eriksson L. Diskectomy of the temporomandibular joint: a double-contrast arthrotomographic follow-up study. Oral Surg Oral Med Oral Pathol 1985;59:435.

34. Hansson L-G, Eriksson L, Westesson P-L. Magnetic resonance evaluation after temporomandibular joint diskectomy. Oral Surg Oral Med Oral Pathol 1992;74:801.

35. Hall HD, Link JL. Diskectomy alone and with ear cartilage interposition grafts in joint reconstruction. Oral Maxillofac Clin North Am 1989;1:329.

36. Dimitroulis G. Condylar morphology after temporomandibular joint discectomy with interpositional abdominal dermis-fat graft. J Oral Maxillofacial Surg 2011;69(2):439–46.

37. Boman K. Temporomandibular joint arthrosis and its treatment by extirpation of the disk: a clinical study. Acta Chir Scand 1947;95:1–154.

38. Laskin DM. Surgical management of internal derangements. In: Laskin DM, Greene CS, Hylander WL, editors. TMDs, an evidence-based approach to diagnosis and treatment. Chicago: Quintessence; 2006. p. 469–81.

39. McKenna SJ. Discectomy for the treatment of internal derangements of the temporomandibular joint. J Oral Maxillofac Surg 2001;59:1051.

40. Hansen WC, Deshazo BW. Siliastic reconstruction of TMJ meniscus. Plast Reconstr Surg 1969;43:4.

41. Dolwick MF, Aufdemorte TB. Silicone induced foreign body reaction and lymphadenopathy after temporomandibular joint arthroplasty. Oral Surg Oral Med Oral Pathol 1985;59:449.

42. Westesson P-L, Eriksson L, Lindstrom C. Destructive lesions of the mandibular condyle following diskectomy with temporary silicone implant. Oral Surg Oral Med Oral Pathol 1987;63:143.

43. Eriksson L, Westesson P-L. Temporomandibular joint discectomy: no positive effect of temporary silicone implant in a 5 year follow-up. Oral Surg Oral Med Oral Pathol 1992;74:259.

44. Keirsch TA: The use of Proplast-Teflon implants for menisectomy and disc repair in the temporomandibular joint. American Association of Oral and Maxillofacial Surgeons Clinical Congress, Program Outlines and Scientific Abstracts, 1984. pp 7–8.

45. Timmis DP, Aragon SB, Van Sickels JE, et al. Comparative study of alloplastic materials for temporomandibular joint disc replacement in rabbits. J Oral Maxillofac Surg 1986;44:451.

46. Heffez L, Mafee MF, Rosenberg H, et al. CT evaluation of temporomandibular disc replacement with a Proplast-Teflon laminate. J Oral Maxillofac Surg 1987;45:657.

47. Food and Drug Administration. TMJ implants: a consumer information update. Rockville (MD): FDA; 1999.

48. Feinberg SE. Use of composite temporalis muscle flaps for disc replacement. Oral Maxillofac Surg Clin North Am 1994;6:335.

49. Smith JA, Sandler NA, Ozaki WH, et al. Subjective and objective assessment of the temporalis myofascial flap in previously operated temporomandibular joints. J Oral Maxillofac Surg 1999;57(9):1058–65 [discussion: 1065–7].

50. Ioannides C, Freihofer PM. Replacement of the damaged interarticular disc of the temporomandibular joint. J Craniomandib Pract 1988;16:273.

51. Tucker MR, Kennady MC, Jacoway JR. Autogenous auricular cartilage implantation following discectomy in the primate temporomandibular joint. J Oral Maxillofac Surg 1990;48:38.

52. Yih W-Y, Zysset M, Merrill RG. Histologic study of the fate of autogenous auricular cartilage grafts in the human temporomandibular joint. J Oral Maxillofac Surg 1992;50:964.

53. Sandler NA, Macmillan C, Buckley MJ, et al. Histologic and histochemical changes in failed auricular cartilage grafts used for a temporomandibular joint disc replacement: a report of 3 cases and review of literature. J Oral Maxillofac Surg 1997;55:1014.

54. Dimitroulis G. The interpositional dermis-fat graft in the management of temporomandibular joint ankylosis. Int J Oral Maxillofac Surg 2004;33(8):755–60.

55. Dimitroulis G, McCullough M, Morrison W. Quality of life survey of patients prior to and following temporomandibular joint discectomy. J Oral Maxillofac Surg 2010;68:101.

56. Candirli C, Demirkol M, Yilmaz O, et al. Retrospective evaluation of three different joint surgeries for internal derangements of the temporomandibular joint. J Craniomaxillofac Surg 2017;45(5):775–80.

57. Kramer, Lee, Beirne. Meta-analysis of TMJ discectomy with or without autogenous/alloplastic interpositional materials: comparative analysis of functional outcome. Int J Oral Maxillofacial Surg 2005;34:69–70.

Costochondral Graft Versus Total Alloplastic Joint for Temporomandibular Joint Reconstruction

Louis G. Mercuri, DDS, MS[a,b,*]

KEYWORDS

- Temporomandibular joint replacement • Costochondral graft • Autogenous bone graft
- Alloplastic temporomandibular replacement

KEY POINTS

- Alloplastic temporomandibular joint (TMJ) replacement devices do not require a donor site.
- Alloplastic TMJ replacement devices require less surgery time.
- Custom alloplastic TMJ replacement devices can be designed and manufactured to conforms to the anatomic situation.
- Alloplastic TMJ replacement device components are not susceptible to prior failed implant foreign body particles or local or systemic pathology.
- Immediately after alloplastic TMJ replacement device implantation, patients can begin physical therapy, hastening regaining mandibular function.

INTRODUCTION

The intricate craniofacial anatomic and functional relationships associated with the temporomandibular joint (TMJ) presents challenges to reconstruction. The function and form of the TMJ is important for mastication, speech, deglutition, airway support, facial esthetics, psychological development, and quality of life.

Considering not only these functional and form issues but also patients' neurologic, physiologic, and biological problems, as well as what can be technically achievable, the following parameters for successful reconstructive outcomes were established (**Box 1**).[1] The indications for TMJ replacement are shown in (**Box 2**).[2] The surgeon presented with any of these scenarios currently has 2 replacement options, either autogenous or alloplastic. This article presents an evidence-based discussion of the advantages and disadvantages of autogenous and alloplastic TMJ replacement to assist both the surgeon and their patients in making that choice.

AUTOGENOUS TEMPOROMANDIBULAR JOINT REPLACEMENT

Autogenous bone grafting has been reported to be the gold standard for the reconstruction of developmental deformities, end-stage TMJ pathology, and ankylosis using either free or vascularized bone grafts from the rib,[3] calvarium,[4] clavicle,[5] iliac crest,[6] or fibula.[7]

Besides the reported unpredictability of autogenous grafting,[8–12] complications frequently arise when transplanting autologous bone.

Disclosure statement: Dr L.G. Mercuri is compensated by TMJ Concepts as a clinical consultant and maintains stock in that company.
[a] Department of Orthopaedic Surgery, Rush University Medical Center, 1611 W Harrison Street, Chicago, IL 60612, USA; [b] TMJ Concepts, 2233 Knoll Drive, Ventura, CA 93003, USA
* TMJ Concepts, 2233 Knoll Drive, Ventura, CA 93003.
E-mail address: lgm@tmjconcepts.com

Oral Maxillofacial Surg Clin N Am 30 (2018) 335–342
https://doi.org/10.1016/j.coms.2018.05.003
1042-3699/18/© 2018 Elsevier Inc. All rights reserved.

Box 1
Parameters for successful temporomandibular joint replacement outcomes

Improvement of mandibular function and form

Reduction of further suffering and disability

Containment of excessive treatment and cost

Prevention of further morbidity

Adapted from Mercuri LG. Alloplastic temporomandibular joint reconstruction. Oral Surg Oral Med Oral Pathol Oral Radiol Endod 1998;85:633; with permission.

Complications associated with iliac crest bone harvest have been reported in up to 19% of cases and include chronic pain, skin sensitivity disorders, and complicated wound healing. These complications can lead to hypertrophic scarring or infection, fracture, and prolonged length of hospitalization, all associated with additional morbidity and medical costs.[13,14]

The costochondral graft has been the most frequently recommended autogenous bone graft for TMJ replacement because of its ease of adaptation to the recipient site, its gross anatomic similarity to the mandibular condyle, the reported low donor site morbidity rate, and its demonstrated growth potential in skeletally immature patients.[3,15–19]

Saeed and Kent[20] reported a retrospective review of 76 costochondral grafts undertaken to determine the outcome with respect to the extent of previous TMJ surgery. The minimum follow-up period was 2 years. The results demonstrated improvement in pain and diet scores, with a moderate increase in interincisal distance. They concluded that in patients with no previous surgery, arthritic disease, or congenital deformity, the costochondral graft performed well. However, a preoperative diagnosis of ankylosis was

---

Box 2
The indications for temporomandibular joint replacement

End-stage arthritic disease

Bony or fibrous ankylosis

Failed autogenous tissue reconstruction

Failed alloplastic reconstruction

Adapted from Mercuri LG, editor. Temporomandibular joint total joint replacement – TMJ TJR – a comprehensive reference for researchers, material scientists and surgeons. New York: Springer; 2015; with permission.

---

associated with a high complication rate and need for further surgery, suggesting caution in that group of patients.

Medra[21] reviewed the records of 55 patients with TMJ ankylosis treated with costochondral grafts followed clinically and radiographically for 7 to 10 years. He reported good remodeling in 59%, reankylosis in 9%, resorption of the graft in 25%, and overgrowth of the graft in 4%. Mouth opening was satisfactory in 58% and unsatisfactory in 18%, and the operation was a failure in 24%.

Reitzik[22] reported that in a situation analogous to autogenous costochondral grafting, cortex-to-cortex healing after vertical ramus osteotomy requires 20 weeks to consolidate in monkeys and probably 25 weeks in humans.

Maxillomandibular fixation (MMF) is typically maintained for some period in patients who have undergone TMJ replacement with costochondral grafts. Despite screw/plate fixation, graft micromotion will invariably occur with any early mandibular function. This micromotion results in shear stresses on the graft/host interface that potentially can lead to poor neovascularization, nonunion, or failure.[23]

The success of any autogenous tissue graft requires the host site have a rich vascular bed. Because of the formation of scar tissue, patients who have undergone multiple surgeries or who have long-standing end-stage TMJ pathology do not provide an environment conducive to the predictable success of free and occasionally vascularized autogenous tissue grafts. Marx[9] reported that capillaries can penetrate a maximum tissue thickness of 180 to 220 μm, whereas scar tissue surrounding previously operated bone averages a thickness of 440 μm. This finding and micromotion may account for the clinical observation that free autogenous tissue bone grafts often fail in those patients who have extreme anatomic architectural discrepancies resulting from prior surgery or pathology.[24]

Theoretically, autogenous costochondral grafts "grow with the patient."[15,17,25] However, often this so-called growth has been reported to be unpredictable or results in ankylosis.[8,26–31] These complications can occur as the result of the micromotion, poor revascularization, or lack of compliance of young patients with postimplantation physical therapy.[32]

Recent studies have even questioned the necessity for using a cartilage-containing graft to restore and maintain mandibular growth.[33,34] Long-term reports of mandibular growth in children whose TMJs were reconstructed with costochondral grafts have demonstrated that excessive growth on the treated side occurred in 54% of the cases examined and growth equal to that on the opposite side occurred in only 38% of the cases.[8–12,35]

In a systematic review of the literature, Kumar and colleagues[36] assessed the growth potential of the costochondral graft for TMJ replacement in patients with ankylosis or hemifacial macrosomia. They concluded that the only evidence was in the form of case series, the lowest level of evidence. Thus, based on available evidence, they concluded that the use of a costochondral graft for TMJ replacement for its growth potential lacks scientific evidence.

In summary, the following are the advantages and disadvantages of using the autogenous costochondral bone graft for TMJ replacement:

Advantages

1. Availability: Ribs are part of every human skeleton. There is no lead time required to purchase and acquire device components; there is no need for an inventory of components, special implantation instruments, or specialized equipment.
2. Biocompatibility: The patients' own bone and cartilage are used; therefore, there are little to no concerns about biocompatibility or hypersensitivity.
3. Adaptability: The graft can be fashioned at surgery to adapt to the form of the lateral surface of the mandible and glenoid fossa.
4. Inexpensive: Alloplastic TMJ replacement components are expensive.

Disadvantages

1. Need for second surgical site: There is increased morbidity and a greater risk of complications.
2. More labor intensive: In some cases, a thoracic or orthopedic surgical team are needed to harvest the graft.
3. Longer surgery: Simultaneous rib harvest and preparation of mandibular implantation sites are most often not feasible, which extends the length of the anesthesia and the surgery.
3. Greater potential for morbidity: Pneumothorax can be a complication of rib harvest. The anesthesia time is longer. Patients may have difficulty with abduction of the ipsilateral upper limb during healing of the donor site.
4. Required bone healing: A costochondral graft is basically a free cortical bone graft, which requires rigid fixation to undergo neovascularization for consolidation into the lateral aspect of the mandible. Research has demonstrated that this requires 20 weeks in monkeys and

probably 25 weeks in humans.[22] Typically, patients with costochondral-grafted TMJ are only kept in MMF a maximum of 4 to 6 weeks. Despite rigid fixation, graft micromotion can occur with early mandibular function, resulting in shear stresses at the graft/host interface that can lead to poor vascularization, nonunion, or potential failure.[23]

5. Delayed physical therapy: Early physical therapy increases the range of motion of reconstructed joints.[37] Keeping patients immobilized (MMF) after any open joint surgery, particularly joint replacement, increases muscle atrophy as well as periarticular fibrosis and the potential for the development of heterotopic ossification and ankylosis.[38]
6. Potential for failure due to the presence of a foreign body reaction or high inflammatory disease: Henry and Wolford[39] demonstrated that the most common cause of failure of autologous tissues placed after failed alloplastic implant removal was fibrous or bony ankylosis. These investigators concluded that the continuation of the foreign body reaction locally long after the implant removal resulted in the failure of the autologous tissue reconstruction. This same principle holds true in cases of high-inflammatory arthritic diseases, such as rheumatoid and psoriatic arthritis.[40]
7. High relapse potential when combined with orthognathic surgery: Restoration of the loss of posterior mandibular height and dental occlusion, as seen in end-stage arthritic disease, condylar resorption, and many cases of obstructive sleep apnea, requires counterclockwise rotation of the mandible along with maxillary surgery in most cases.[41] This maneuver places great stress on the costochondral graft. Relapse has been reported to be high when autogenous costochondral grafting has been used to reconstruct the condyle in such cases.[42–44]

ALLOPLASTIC TEMPOROMANDIBULAR JOINT REPLACEMENT

Because of the various disadvantages of autogenous costochondral grafting, there arose the need for the development of alloplastic materials to replace the anatomically and functionally impaired TMJ. This course is similar to the course followed by orthopedic surgery in replacement of other end-stage diseased body joints.[2]

In 1995, Chase and colleagues[45] reported the use of a thin cast Vitallium fossa-eminence hemi-arthroplasty prosthesis for management of TMJ ankylosis (Christensen prosthesis). A cast Vitallium ramus-condyle component with a polymethylmethacrylate head was later added to create a total joint prosthesis (**Fig. 1**). Because of the wear under functional loading,[46] this bearing surface was abandoned in the late 1990s for a metal-on-metal bearing surface.[47] This metal-metal device was marketed by Nexus CMF (Salt Lake City, UT) until 2017.

In 1993, Kent and colleagues[48] reported on the long-term follow-up of the Vitek (Houston, TX) partial and total TMJ reconstruction prostheses (**Fig. 2**). With the subsequent publications on the material failure and complications with Proplast-polytetrafluoroethylene (Teflon), the need for an improved alloplastic TMJ replacement system grew. Van Loon and colleagues[49] and Driemel and colleagues[50] have reviewed much of the early history of the development, utilization, and outcomes of the various TMJ total joint replacement (TJR) devices.

In 1995, Mercuri and colleagues[51] reported on preliminary results with the use of the Techmedica

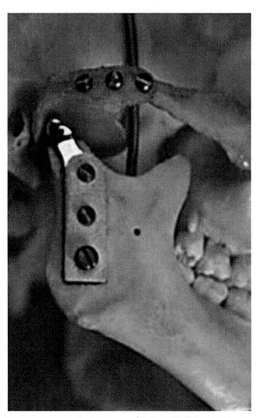

Fig. 2. Kent-Vitek (Houston, TX) total TMJ reconstruction prostheses. (*Modified from* Quinn PD, Granquist EJ. Atlas of temporomandibular joint surgery. Ames (IA): Wiley Blackwell; 2015. p. 152; with permission.)

(Camarillo, CA) patient-fitted (custom) computer-assisted designed (CAD)/computer-assisted manufactured (CAM) total alloplastic TMJ reconstruction prosthesis in a prospective limited clinical study (**Fig. 3**). Based on this study, TMJ Concepts (Ventura, CA) received approval from the Food and Drug Administration (FDA) to manufacture and market this device in 1999.[52] Since that time 10-, 14-, and 20-year follow-up studies[53–55] have been reported demonstrating the safety and efficacy of this device (**Fig. 4**).

In 2000, Quinn[55] introduced the stock Biomet Microfixation (Jacksonville, FL) TMJ TJR device.[56] This system received FDA approval to be manufactured and marketed based on a clinical study published later by Giannakopoulos and colleagues.[56] Further long-term studies using this device have been reported.[57–66]

The results of studies comparing the currently available FDA-approved alloplastic total TMJ replacement systems support the use of both stock and custom systems. Further, these studies demonstrate that alloplastic total TMJ replacement is safe and effective, reduces pain, improves

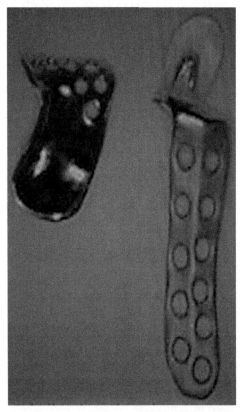

Fig. 1. Christensen (TMJ, Inc, Golden, CO) cast Vitallium fossa and ramus-condyle component with a polymethylmethacrylate head. (*Modified from* Quinn PD, editor. Color atlas of temporomandibular joint surgery. St Louis (MO): Mosby; 1998. p. 190; with permission.)

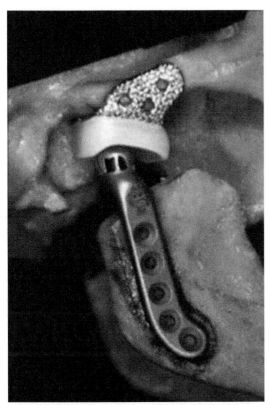

Fig. 3. Techmedica (Camarillo, CA) patient-fitted CAD/CAM total alloplastic TMJ reconstruction prosthesis. (*Courtesy of* TMJ Concepts, Ventura, CA.)

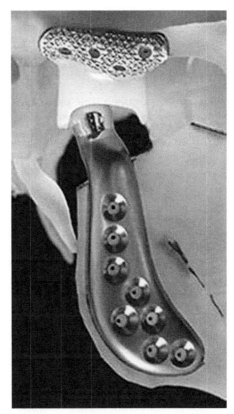

Fig. 4. TMJ Concepts (Ventura, CA) patient-fitted CAD/CAM total alloplastic TMJ reconstruction prosthesis. (*Courtesy of* TMJ Concepts, Ventura, CA.)

mandibular function and patients' quality of life, and has few complications. Therefore, these devices represent a viable and stable long-term solution for TMJ reconstruction in patients with irreversible end-stage disease.[60–67]

Lee and colleagues[68] have reviewed the published research that compared the outcomes of autogenous costochondral grafting and alloplastic TMJ reconstruction. Using the PubMed database and including prospective, retrospective, case-control, and longitudinal studies, and with significant statistical analysis, these investigators divided outcomes into acceptable or nonacceptable. They discovered 7 articles that dealt with costochondral grafting in 180 patients. Most patients had good outcomes (n = 109, 61%). They found 6 articles with 275 patients who had undergone alloplastic TMJ replacements. These patients had excellent outcomes (n = 261, 95%). The investigators concluded that alloplastic total joint reconstruction resulted in increased quality of life and fewer complications compared with autogenous costochondral grafting. Therefore, alloplastic TMJ replacement was deemed more effective for total joint replacement than costochondral grafting.[69–73]

The following is a summary of the advantages and disadvantages associated with alloplastic TMJ replacement:

Advantages

1. Availability: Stock systems can be inventoried and immediately available for use, as needed.
2. There is no donor site morbidity.
3. Decreased surgery time: no donor site is involved.
4. Conforms to the anatomic situation: A custom system provides components that are designed and manufactured to fit exactly with the specific anatomy.
5. Components are not susceptible to foreign body particles from prior failed prostheses or high inflammatory pathology.
6. Patients can begin physical therapy immediately.

Disadvantages

1. Expense: Although the operating room, anesthesia, and surgical time charges are much less than with autogenous costochondral graft harvest and implantation, the total cost of

alloplastic TMJ replacement is at least comparable or may be less.

2. Longevity of the components: Current studies indicate that alloplastic TMJ replacement devices have a lifespan of at least 10 to 20 years.[54,57]

3. Material hypersensitivity: The percentage of aseptic failures due to biomaterial hypersensitivity in alloplastic TMJ replacement is unknown.[69]

4. Currently, it is only indicated for skeletally mature patients.

SUMMARY

Based on the evidence cited, alloplastic TMJ replacement seems to provide the most predictable functional and esthetic outcomes in patients with end-stage TMJ disease.

REFERENCES

1. Mercuri LG. Alloplastic temporomandibular joint reconstruction. Oral Surg Oral Med Oral Oral Pathol Oral Radiol Endod 1998;85:631–7.

2. Mercuri LG, editor. Temporomandibular joint total joint replacement – TMJ TJR – a comprehensive reference for researchers, material scientists and surgeons. New York: Springer International Publishing; 2015.

3. MacIntosh RB. The use of autogenous tissue in temporomandibular joint reconstruction. J Oral Maxillofac Surg 2000;58:63–9.

4. Lee JJ, Worthington P. Reconstruction of the temporomandibular joint using calvarial bone after a failed Teflon-Proplast implant. J Oral Maxillofac Surg 1999;57:457–61.

5. Wolford LM, Cottrell DA, Henry C. Sternoclavicular grafts for temporomandibular joint reconstruction. J Oral Maxillofac Surg 1994;52:119–28.

6. Kummoona R. Chondro-osseous iliac crest graft for one stage reconstruction of the ankylosed TMJ in children. J Maxillofac Surg 1986;14:215–20.

7. Fariña R, Campos P, Beytía J, et al. Reconstruction of Temporomandibular Joint with a Fibula Free Flap: A Case Report with a Histological Study. J Oral Maxillofac Surg 2015;73:2449.e1-5.

8. Guyuron B, Lasa CI. Unpredictable growth pattern of costochondral graft. Plast Reconstr Surg 1992;90:880–6.

9. Marx RE. The science and art of reconstructing the jaws and temporomandibular joints. In: Bell WH, editor. Modern practice in orthognathic and reconstructive surgery, vol. 2. Philadelphia: Saunders; 1992. p. 1448–531.

10. Svensson A, Adell R. Costochondral grafts to replace mandibular condyles in juvenile chronic arthritis patients: Long-term effects on facial growth. J Craniomaxillofac Surg 1998;26:275–85.

11. Ross RB. Costochondral grafts replacing the mandibular condyle. Cleft Palate Craniofac J 1999;36:334–9.

12. Wen-Ching K, Huang C-S, Chen Y-R. Temporomandibular joint reconstruction in children using costochondral grafts. J Oral Maxillofac Surg 1999;57:789–98.

13. Dimitroulis G. Temporomandibular joint surgery: what does it mean to the dental practitioner? Aust Dent J 2011;56:257–64.

14. Nkenke E, Neukam FW. Autogenous bone harvesting and grafting in advanced jaw resorption: morbidity, resorption and implant survival. Eur J Oral Implantol 2014;7(Suppl 2):S203–17.

15. Ware WH, Taylor RC. Cartilaginous growth centers transplanted to replace mandibular condyles in monkeys. J Oral Surg 1966;24:33–43.

16. Poswillo DE. Experimental reconstruction of the mandibular joint. Int J Oral Surg 1974;3:400–11.

17. Ware WH, Brown SL. Growth center transplantation to replace mandibular condyles. J Maxillofac Surg 1981;9:50–8.

18. MacIntosh RB. Current spectrum of costochondral grafting. In, surgical correction of dentofacial deformities. In: Bell WH, editor. New concepts, vol. III. Philadelphia: Saunders; 1985. p. 355–410.

19. Poswillo DE. Biological reconstruction of the mandibular condyle. Br J Oral Maxillofac Surg 1987;25:100–4.

20. Saeed NR, Kent JN. A retrospective study of the costochondral graft in TMJ reconstruction. Int J Oral Maxillofac Surg 2003;32:606–9.

21. Medra AM. Follow up of mandibular costochondral grafts after release of ankylosis of the temporomandibular joints. Br J Oral Maxillofac Surg 2005;43:118–22.

22. Reitzik M. Cortex-to-cortex healing after mandibular osteotomy. J Oral Maxillofac Surg 1983;41:658–63.

23. Lienau J, Schell H, Duda G. Initial vascularization and tissue differentiation are influenced by fixation stability. J Orthop Res 2005;23:639–45.

24. Mercuri LG. The use of alloplastic prostheses for temporomandibular joint reconstruction. J Oral Maxillofac Surg 2000;58:70–5.

25. MacIntosh RB, Henny FA. A spectrum of application of autogenous costochondral grafts. J Maxillofac Surg 1977;5:257–67.

26. Samman N, Cheung LK, Tideman H. Overgrowth of a costochondral graft in an adult male. Int J Oral Maxillofac Surg 1995;24:333–5.

27. Esguep-Sarah A, Chaparro-Padilla A, Quevedo-Rojas L. Histopathologic study of costochondral graft with overgrowth functioning as mandibular condyle. Med Oral 1997;2:140–5.

28. Baek RM, Song YT. Overgrowth of a costochondral graft in reconstruction of the temporomandibular joint. Scand J Plast Reconstr Surg Hand Surg 2006;40:179–85.

29. Siavosh S, Ali M. Overgrowth of a costochondral graft in a case of temporomandibular joint ankylosis. J Craniofac Surg 2007;18:1488–91.

30. Yang S, Fan H, Du W, et al. Overgrowth of costochondral grafts in craniomaxillofacial reconstruction: Rare complication and literature review. J Craniomaxillofac Surg 2015;43:803–12.

31. Razzak A, Ahmed N, Sidebottom A. Management of facial asymmetry due to overgrowing costochondral graft: a case report. Int J Surg Case Rep 2016;26: 93–5.

32. Mercuri LG, Swift JQ. Considerations for the use of alloplastic temporomandibular joint replacement in the growing patient. J Oral Maxillofac Surg 2009; 67:1979–90.

33. Ellis E, Schneiderman ED, Carlson DS. Growth of the mandible after replacement of the mandibular condyle: an experimental investigation in Macaca mulatta. J Oral Maxillofac Surg 2002;60:1461–70.

34. Guyot L, Richard O, Layoun W, et al. Long-term radiological findings following reconstruction of the condyle with fibular free flaps. J Craniomaxillofac Surg 2004;32:98–102.

35. Perrot DH, Umeda H, Kaban LB. Costochondral graft/reconstruction of the condyle/ramus unit: long-term follow-up. Int J Oral Maxillofac Surg 1994;23:321–8.

36. Kumar P, Rattan V, Rai S. Do costochondral grafts have any growth potential in temporomandibular joint surgery? A systematic review. J Oral Biol Craniofac Res 2015;5:198–202.

37. Salter RB. The biologic concept of continuous passive motion of synovial joints. The first 18 years of basic research and its clinical application. Clin Orthop Relat Res 1989;242:12–25.

38. Mercuri LG, Saltzman BM. Acquired heterotopic ossification in alloplastic joint replacement. Int J Oral Maxillofac Surg 2017;46:1562–8.

39. Henry CH, Wolford LM. Treatment outcomes for temporomandibular joint reconstruction after Proplast-Teflon implant failure. J Oral Maxillofac Surg 1993;51:352–8.

40. Mercuri LG. Surgical management of TMJ arthritis. In: Laskin DM, Greene CS, Hylander WL, editors. Temporomandibular joint disorders: an evidence-based approach to diagnosis and treatment. Chicago: Quintessence; 2006. p. 455–68.

41. Al-Moraissi EA, Wolford LM. Is counterclockwise rotation of the maxillomandibular complex stable compared with clockwise rotation in the correction of dentofacial deformities? A systematic review and meta-analysis. J Oral Maxillofac Surg 2016;74: 2066.e1–12.

42. Crawford JG, Stoelinga PJ, Blijdorp PA, et al. Stability after reoperation of progressive condylar resorption after orthognathic surgery. J Oral Maxillofac Surg 1994;52:460–6.

43. Huang YL, Ross BR. Diagnosis and management of condylar resorption. J Oral Maxillofac Surg 1997;55: 114–9.

44. Hoppenreijs TJM, Stoelinga PJ, Grace KL, et al. Long-term evaluation of patients with progressive condylar resorption following orthognathic surgery. Int J Oral Maxillofac Surg 1999;28:411–8.

45. Chase DC, Hudson JW, Gerard DA, et al. The christensen prosthesis. Oral Surg 1995;80:273–8.

46. Mercuri LG. The Christensen prosthesis. Oral Surg Oral Med Oral Pathol Oral Radiol Endod 1996;81: 134–5.

47. Lippincott AL III, Dowling JM, Phil D, et al. Temporomandibular joint arthroplasty using metal-on-metal and acrylic-on-metal configurations: wear in laboratory tests and in retrievals. Surg Technol Int 1999;8: 321–30.

48. Kent JN, Block MS, Halpern J, et al. Long-term results on VK partial and total temporomandibular joint systems. J Long Term Eff Med Implants 1993;3:29–40.

49. Van Loon JP, DeBont LGM, Boering G. Evaluation of temporomandibular joint prostheses: Review of the literature from 1946 -1994 and implications for future designs. J Oral Maxillofac Surg 1995;53:984–96.

50. Driemel O, Braun S, Müller-Richter UD, et al. Historical development of alloplastic temporomandibular joint replacement after 1945 and state of the art. Int J Oral Maxillofac Surg 2009;38:909–20.

51. Mercuri LG, Wolford LM, Sanders B, et al. Custom CAD/CAM total temporomandibular joint reconstruction system: preliminary multicenter report. J Oral Maxillofac Surg 1995;53:106–15.

52. Mercuri LG, Wolford LM, Sanders B, et al. Long-term follow-up of the CAD/CAM patient-fitted total temporomandibular joint reconstruction system. J Oral Maxillofac Surg 2002;60:1440–8.

53. Mercuri LG, Edibam NR, Giobbie-Hurder A. 14-year follow-up of a patient fitted total temporomandibular joint reconstruction system. J Oral Maxillofac Surg 2007;65:1140–8.

54. Wolford LM, Mercuri LG, Schneiderman ED, et al. Twenty-year follow-up study on a patient-fitted temporomandibular joint prosthesis: the techmedica/TMJ concepts device. J Oral Maxillofac Surg 2015;73:952–60.

55. Quinn PD. Lorenz prosthesis. In: Total temporomandibular joint reconstruction. Donlon WC, editor. Oral and Maxillofac Surgery Clinics of North America (series);12:93–104.

56. Giannakopoulos HE, Sinn DP, Quinn PD. Biomet microfixation temporomandibular joint replacement system: a 3-year follow-up study of patients treated

during 1995 to 2005. J Oral Maxillofac Surg 2012;70: 787–94.

57. Leandro LF, Ono HY, Loureiro CC, et al. A ten-year experience and follow-up of three hundred patients fitted with the Biomet/Lorenz Microfixation TMJ replacement system. Int J Oral Maxillofac Surg 2013;42:1007–13.

58. Sanovich R, Mehta U, Abramowicz S, et al. Total allo-plastic temporomandibular joint reconstruction us-ing Biomet stock prostheses: the University of Florida experience. Int J Oral Maxillofac Surg 2014;43:1091–5.

59. Aagaard E, Thygesen T. A prospective, single-centre study on patient outcomes following temporo-mandibular joint replacement using a custom-made Biomet TMJ prosthesis. Int J Oral Maxillofac Surg 2014;43:1229–35.

60. Wolford LM, Dingwerth DJ, Talwar RM, et al. Com-parison of two temporomandibular joint total joint prosthesis systems. J Oral Maxillofac Surg 2003; 61:685–90.

61. Guarda-Nardini L, Manfredini D, Ferronato G. Temporomandibular joint total replacement pros-thesis: current knowledge and considerations for the future. Int J Oral Maxillofac Surg 2008;37: 103–10.

62. Al-Moraissi EA, El-Sharkawy TM, Mounair RM, et al. A systematic review and meta-analysis of the clinical outcomes for various surgical modalities in the man-agement of temporomandibular joint ankylosis. Int J Oral Maxillofac Surg 2015;44:470–82.

63. Zieman MT, McKenzie WS, Louis PJ. Comparison of temporomandibular joint reconstruction with custom (TMJ Concepts) vs. stock (Biomet) prostheses. J Oral Maxillofac Surg 2015;(Supplement 73):e79.

64. Gonzalez-Perez LM, Gonzalez-Perez-Somarriba B, Centeno G, et al. Evaluation of total alloplastic temporomandibular joint replacement with two different types of prostheses: a three-year prospec-tive study. Med Oral Patol Oral Cir Bucal 2016;21: e766–75.

65. Kunjur J, Niziol R, Matthews NS. Quality of life: patient-reported outcomes after total replacement of the temporomandibular joint. Br J Oral Maxillofac Surg 2016;54:762–6.

66. Wojczyńska A, Leiggener CS, Bredell M, et al. Allo-plastic total temporomandibular joint replacements: do they perform like natural joints? Prospective cohort study with a historical control. Int J Oral Max-illofac Surg 2016;45:1213–21.

67. Johnson NR, Roberts MJ, Doi SA, et al. Total TMJ replacement prostheses: a systematic review and bias-adjusted meta-analysis. Int J Oral Maxillofac Surg 2017;46:86–92.

68. Lee WY, Park YW, Kim SG. Comparison of costo-chondral graft and customized total joint reconstruc-tion for treatments of temporomandibular joint replacement. Maxillofac Plast Reconstr Surg 2014; 36:135–9.

69. Hallab NJ. Material hypersensitivity. In: Mercuri LG, editor. Temporomandibular joint total joint replace-ment – TMJ TJR – a comprehensive reference for re-searchers, material scientists and surgeons. New York: Springer International Publishing; 2016. p. 227–50.

70. Banda AK, Chopra K, Keyser B, et al. Alloplastic to-tal temporomandibular joint replacement in skele-tally immature patients: a pilot survey. Proceedings of the Annual Scientific Session American Society of TMJ Surgeons. Miami, FL, March 6, 2015.

71. Moss ML, Salentijn L. The capsular matrix. Am J Or-thod 1969;56:474–90.

72. Moss ML. Twenty years of functional cranial anal-ysis. Am J Orthod 1972;61:479–85.

73. Moss ML. Functional cranial analysis and the func-tional matrix. Int J Orthod 1979;17:21–31.

Injectable Agents Versus Surgery for Recurrent Temporomandibular Joint Dislocation

Shravan Kumar Renapurkar, BDS, DMD,
Daniel M. Laskin, DDS, MS*

KEYWORDS

- Temporomandibular joint dislocation • Subluxation • Eminectomy • Autologous blood injection
- Sclerosing agents

KEY POINTS

- Recurrent temporomandibular joint dislocation is a challenging entity in clinical practice and type of dislocation is a major determinant of the type of treatment.
- There is a lack of high-level evidence to support the superiority of one surgical technique over the other.
- Surgical treatments seem to work secondary to periarticular or intra-articular scarring causing reduced hypermobility.
- Minimally invasive injectable agents show promising results, with low risk, compared with surgical techniques hence they should be the initial treatment for recurrent mandibular dislocation.
- Capsulorraphy and/or eminectomy can be the next best approach for treatment.

INTRODUCTION

Recurrent temporomandibular joint dislocation (TMJD), although relatively uncommon, presents a treatment challenge for the oral and maxillofacial surgeon. Use of a variety of terms interchangeably, such as open lock, dislocation, luxation, subluxation, and hypermobility, along with a lack of clear evidence in the literature supporting its management, adds to the dilemma.[1] Two major current techniques include the injectable agents and surgical techniques, each having their own pros and cons, indications, and reported efficacy. This article critically evaluates the current literature and provides evidence-based recommendations regarding the use of these techniques.

PATHOGENESIS AND CLASSIFICATION OF TEMPOROMANDIBULAR JOINT DISLOCATION

When the mandibular condyle is located anterior to the glenoid fossa and anterior-superior to the articular eminence while in translation, but is self-reducible by the patient, it is termed a subluxation. A true TMJD, by contrast, is not self-reducible and commonly requires an intervention under either local or general anesthesia to return the condyle to the fossa (**Fig. 1**).[2]

TMJD is commonly classified into acute and chronic recurrent types.[3–5] Acute TMJD is more common and can occur secondary to facial trauma, prolonged dental procedures, and endotracheal intubation. The pathogenesis of recurrent

Disclosure: The authors have nothing to disclose.
Department of Oral and Maxillofacial Surgery, Virginia Commonwealth University, 520 North 12th Street, Wood Building Room 311C, Richmond, VA 23298, USA
* Corresponding author.
E-mail address: dmlaskin@vcu.edu

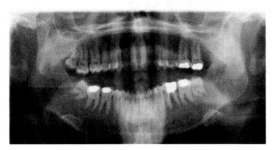

Fig. 1. Panoramic radiograph showing bilateral TMJD.

TMJ dislocation is as controversial as its treatment. Although the exact etiology of TMJD is unknown, it is reported to be multifactorial.[6] Some investigators support a soft tissue abnormality in its pathogenesis, such as laxity of the capsule/ligaments, whereas others relate it to an abnormality in the bony anatomy (eminence/fossa, condyle).[7–10] In either case, an anatomic abnormality has been considered to be a factor precipitating instability of the joint and resulting in dislocation. Chronic recurrent TMJD also can be associated with neuromuscular conditions, medications used in treatment of psychiatric disorders, seizures, and connective tissue disorders like Ehlers-Danlos syndrome.[11–16] Positioning of the mandibular condyle anterior to the TMJ disc has also been suggested to be a cause of pseudo-TMJD.[17]

MANAGEMENT OF TEMPOROMANDIBULAR JOINT DISLOCATION

The type of dislocation is a major determinant of the method of management chosen. Acute dislocation can be managed with immediate manual reduction under local or general anesthesia. Following reduction, a short period of restricted jaw motion has been recommended, combined with use of a muscle relaxant medication.

If an acute dislocation continues to recur, it becomes the chronic recurrent type. Although it can still be immediately reduced under local or general anesthesia, it warrants an adjunctive intervention aimed at eliminating the chance of recurrence. This involves either a minimally invasive procedure using injectable agents aimed at producing histologic changes in the periarticular soft tissues or open surgical procedures aimed at manipulating the periarticular soft tissues, the hard tissues, or both.

Acute dislocation, if left untreated for any reason, can progress to a long-standing/chronic protracted stage. Reduction of long-standing TMJD, even under general anesthesia, becomes more difficult with time and conservative management generally does not have predictable success.[18] There are various techniques reported to reduce prolonged or long-standing TMJD, almost all performed under general anesthesia.[19]

The specific treatment chosen for management of acute and chronic TMJD should be based on proven efficacy. The following is a discussion of the findings from the literature regarding this issue.

Injectable Agents

The advantages and disadvantages of injectable agents are outlined in **Box 1**. The basis for using injectable agents lies in their ability to induce fibrosis of the capsular and periarticular tissues, which in turn reduces translation of the condyle and hence prevents dislocation. There are several injectable agents reported in the literature with varying success rates. Commonly used agents include sclerosing agents, autologous blood, and Botulinum toxin (BTX) A.

Sclerosing agents (chemical capsulorraphy)

Sclerosing agents were of significant interest when Hacker first published on alcohol injections in 1884.[20] Since then, various other agents have

---

Box 1
Advantages and disadvantages of injectable agents for treatment of temporomandibular joint dislocation

Advantages

1. Least-invasive procedure
2. Can be performed in an outpatient office setting
3. Agents easy to obtain
4. Low cost compared with surgical interventions
5. Little chance of serious morbidity, such as facial nerve injury
6. Easy learning curve
7. Quick procedure

Disadvantages

1. Repeated injections may be needed
2. Off-label use
3. Lack of data on long-term follow-up
4. Lack of data on long-term effects on articular cartilage

been used in treatment of recurrent TMJD. Schultz[21] in 1947 described the injection of sodium psylliate into the periarticular tissues to limit translation by inducing fibrosis. His study involved both animal interventions to confirm safety, followed by clinical application in 30 patients with a high success rate. However, length of follow-up and recurrence rates were not quantified. The reported success rate in later reports was approximately 72% to 75%.[5,7]

In more recent years, prolotherapy or "regenerative injection therapy" has gained interest. It had been used for several indications, including arthritic and inflammatory conditions of the axial joints over the past century. It is based on the presumption that the proliferative agent creates a low-grade inflammatory response in the tissues that promotes growth factor activity resulting in repair and regeneration of the tissues. The most common proliferative agent used is dextrose in varying concentrations (10%–50%).[22,23] The few prospective, randomized clinical studies reported with use of dextrose injections show significantly reduced pain but an ambiguous response to joint range of motion when compared with placebo injections.[24,25] It has been proposed that the response could be secondary to the needle trauma rather than the dextrose itself. Irrespective of the type of injectable agent used, multiple injections are sometimes needed to gain improvement in symptoms.

Autologous blood

Autologous blood injection (ABI) for the treatment of recurrent TMJD was first reported by Brachmann in 1964.[26] Injection of autologous blood carries the advantages of being inexpensive and easy to obtain without any special equipment. Most articles describe an injection technique similar to TMJ arthrocentesis, with or without a short course of postoperative maxillomandibular fixation (MMF). The principle behind use of autologous blood is based on the pathogenesis of posttraumatic hemarthrosis, with its subsequent scarring and limitation in range of motion of the condyle.[27]

ABI when combined with MMF has been reported to be more effective than ABI alone in reducing recurrence of TMJD and limiting range of motion of the mandible.[28] In general, the success rate with limited follow-up has been reported to be approximately 60% to 80%.[29] Due to similarity in the formation of a fibrous ankylosis in some patients with posttraumatic hemarthrosis, there are concerns about the long-term effect of ABI into the joint

space. However, in a study supported by preoperative and postoperative MRIs on patients who received ABI for TMJD, there was no evidence of fibrosis or articular changes after 4 weeks.[30] On the other hand, there have been conflicting results in animal studies on the effects of blood being in contact with cartilage.[31–34] None of the clinical reports have reported any serious consequences, but there is lack of long-term data.

Botulinum toxin

Injection of BTX for chronic recurrent dislocation is based on the theory that the lateral pterygoid muscle when hyperactive contributes to the dislocation of the TMJ. A subset of patients who have neurologic disorders, such as multiple sclerosis, Parkinson disease, or cerebral palsy, are reported to have a muscular imbalance sometimes resulting in "neurogenic" TMJD.[35] Once injected in therapeutic doses, BTX weakens the lateral pterygoid muscle by inhibiting acetylcholine release in the synaptic cleft, which decreases its activity and prevents dislocation.[35,36] Anywhere between 25 and 100 units of BTX-A (commonly used type of BTX) have been used for the injections.[37–39] Injection of BTX into the inferior belly of the lateral pterygoid muscle, which attaches to the neck of the condyle, is described using either an extraoral or intraoral approach, with or without electromyographic guidance or preinjection anatomic measurements on a computed tomography scan.[39,40] Although BTX injection has been reported to be effective in management of TMJD even after a single injection, most articles report the need for multiple injections until attaining the desired clinical effect because its action lasts for only 2 to 4 months.

Use of BTX for TMJD is off-label and all the studies supporting its efficacy have either a limited number of patients and/or a follow-up time of only 8 months to 2 years. There has been no prospective clinical trial reported. Risk of diffusion of BTX into adjacent or deeper musculature resulting in, for example, dysphagia, nasal regurgitation, or facial nerve weakness, exists, but is rare and transient (2–4 weeks).[40]

Surgical Interventions

As opposed to injectable agent techniques, surgical approaches involve elaborate preparation, incorporate a longer learning curve, and inherently involve procedural risks. There are several surgical interventions described in the past century that are claimed to be reliable. These interventions either aim to create an obstruction to, or restriction of, condylar translation to prevent dislocation, or they remove the articular eminence, which is presumed to prevent the condyle from returning back into the glenoid fossa.

Capsulorrhaphy

Tightening or strengthening of the TMJ capsule and ligaments is based on the concept that ligamentous or capsular laxity is a cause or precipitating factor in TMJD.[5] Capsulorraphy has been described using an arthrotomy approach as well as with an arthroscopic technique. The arthroscopic technique is fairly recent and involves use of adjunctive sclerosing agents, a laser, and/or electrocautery.[41,42] Arthroscopic techniques aim to create scarring in the oblique protuberance or the retrodiscal region of the joint capsule. This technique is minimally invasive, and caries lower morbidity and risks compared with open techniques. The success rates with arthroscopic capsulorraphy have been reported to be between 82% and 95%.[42,43]

Open capsulorraphy techniques, in contrast to arthroscopic techniques, aim to directly tighten the capsule and ligaments. Although reported to be successful, the studies on capsulorraphy have similar limitations of low number of subjects and varying follow-up periods as those involving nonsurgical methods.[44–46]

Eminectomy

Eminectomy was first described by Myrhaug[9] in 1951 based on radiographic studies showing steepness in the eminences of patients with recurrent TMJD, which was then considered to be the barrier preventing return of a dislocated condyle into the fossa. It involves surgical reduction of the articular eminence, typically performed via a preauricular or endaural approach. In general, eminectomy has been reported to have a 72% to 100% rate of success in eliminating recurrence of dislocation.

Although it is claimed that the success of eminectomy is based on the idea that the articular eminence prevents an anteriorly positioned condyle from returning to the glenoid fossa, this concept is not supported by a consideration of the regional anatomy. The area anterior to the eminence, the preglenoid plane, is flat and therefore cannot act as an obstruction. Rather, the effectiveness of eminectomy is based on postoperative scarring in the joint and not removal of the eminence.[20]

LeClerc procedure/Dautrey procedure

This procedure, aimed at creating interference in the condylar translation path by using a displaced segment of the zygomatic arch, was first described by Mayer[47] in 1933. LeClerc and Girard[48] described a variation of this technique by making a vertical osteotomy in the zygomatic arch and inferiorly positioning the proximal side to alter the condylar path. Gosserez and Dautrey in 1967 modified the technique wherein they made the osteotomy of the zygomatic arch in an oblique fashion angled anterio-inferiorly, along with a green stick fracture of the zygomatico-temporal suture, followed by medial and inferior inset of the osteotomized side under the eminence.[49] This technique, now commonly known as the "Dautrey procedure," has been reported in several studies. Success rates with this technique have been acceptable and vary between 67% and 100%.[50–55] Concern over resorption of the zygomatic fragment, inadvertent complete fracture of the anterior portion of the arch requiring fixation, and failure due to lateral placement of the bony segment have all been reported.[55–58] Fixation of the proximal side using hardware to maintain the desired medial position has been recommended.[52]

Augmentation procedures

Augmentation procedures aim to create an obstruction or a blockade to the condylar translation path using various materials, such as an autogenous bone graft or alloplastic materials. The calvarium and iliac crest are commonly used autogenous sources of bone.[59] An osteotomy is created in the eminence, which is then down fractured while keeping the medial periosteum intact. The bone graft or alloplastic material is then placed in the osteotomy to augment the height of eminence and secured with wire or a plate. The overall success rate for this procedure is deemed to be approximately 65% to 100%.[59–61]

Lateral pterygoid myotomy

The basis for lateral pterygoid myotomy is to detach the muscle that is responsible for anterior translation of the condyle. This, in turn, reduces the chance of TMJD because it limits translation. Lateral pterygoid myotomy has been described via both intraoral and extraoral approaches, but the data are limited and without long-term follow-up.[62,63] There have been no recent studies on this procedure. Temporalis myotomy has been advocated by Laskin[64] for protracted dislocations on the basis that spasticity or fibrosis of the temporalis muscle prevents the condyle from returning to the fossa.

DISCUSSION

As with most of the literature in oral and maxillofacial surgery, the evidence supporting treatments for recurrent TMJD is level 4 per the Center for Evidence-based Medicine criteria. There are only a few prospective randomized clinical trials supporting injectable agent-based treatment and they have relatively few subjects and short follow-up periods. There are no level I evidence studies supporting the surgical treatment options. As with any irreversible invasive surgical procedure, there are several ethical and logistical challenges to conducting a randomized double-blind clinical trial on TMJ surgery; hence, such information may never be available. Therefore, clinical decisions have to be made based on the best available evidence.

Current Evidence for Injectable Agents

Currently, there has been renewed interest and a large amount of literature supporting injectable agents and their efficacy. A recent prospective randomized clinical trial involving 48 patients compared ABI alone versus MMF alone versus ABI + MMF.[28] Although the group with ABI alone required multiple injections before lack of recurrence, the study reported no recurrence of TMJD when ABI was combined with 4 weeks of maxillomandibular fixation in up to 80% of patients. Based on such findings, use of an injectable agent is recommended as the initial treatment of patients with TMJD.

Current Evidence for Surgical Treatment

The current literature shows variable success rates for surgical treatment of TMJD. Due to heterogeneity in the study samples and other variables affecting the rate of recurrence, it is difficult to conclude what is the best available surgical option. However, there is one commonality among most of the procedures that can help in making this decision: most of the operations are intracapsular and result in postoperative fibrosis and scarring in the joint that limits jaw movement. On this basis, capsulorraphy appears to be the most logical initial surgical operation because it is minimally invasive and has fewer risks than the other possible procedures. Failure of such an option would then warrant one of the other more invasive surgical procedures. Of these, eminectomy is probably the most favorable.

SUMMARY

Pathophysiology, medical history, and the type or variant of TMJD have a crucial role in determining the type of treatment selected. Patients with acute dislocation should be managed with immediate reduction and a short period of jaw motion restriction with or without MMF. If dislocation becomes recurrent, a minimally invasive approach using an injectable agent, such as autologous blood or a sclerosing agent, should be the method of choice. Failing this minimally invasive intervention, an open surgical approach can be used. Of those available, capsulorraphy is the most logical because it is least invasive and has fewer potential risks. In unresponsive patients, eminectomy is recommended.

REFERENCES

1. Melo AR, Pereira Júnior ED, Santos LAM, et al. Recurrent dislocation: scientific evidence and management following a systematic review. Int J Oral Maxillofac Surg 2017;46(7):851–6.
2. Nitzan D. Temporomandibular joint "open lock" versus condylar dislocation: signs and symptoms, imaging, treatment, and pathogenesis. J Oral Maxillofac Surg 2002;60:506–11.
3. Adekeye EO, Shamia RI, Cove P. Inverted L-shaped ramus osteotomy for prolonged bilateral dislocation of the temporomandibular joint. Oral Surg Oral Med Oral Pathol 1976;41:568–77.
4. Rowe NL, Killey HC. Fractures of the facial skeleton. 2nd edition. Edinburgh (Scotland): E & S Livingstone; 1970. p. 23–34.
5. Shorey CW, Campbell JH. Dislocation of the temporomandibular joint. Oral Surg Oral Med Oral Pathol Oral Radiol Endod 2000;89:662–8.
6. Liddell A, Perez DE. Temporomandibular joint dislocation. Oral Maxillofac Surg Clin North Am 2015; 27(1):125–36.
7. McKelvey LE. Sclerosing solution in the treatment of chronic subluxation of the temporomandibular joint. J Oral Surg 1950;8:225–36.
8. Schultz LW. Report of ten years' experience in treating hypermobility of the temporomandibular joint. J Oral Surg 1947;5:202–7.
9. Myrhaug H. New method of operation for habitual dislocation of mandible. Acta Odontol Scand 1951; 9:247–61.
10. Leopard PJ. Surgery of the non-ankylosed temporomandibular joint. Br J Oral Maxillofac Surg 1987;25: 138–48.
11. O'Connor M, Rooney M, Nienaber CP. Neuroleptic-induced dislocation of the jaw. Br J Psychiatry 1992;161:281.
12. Wood GD. An adverse reaction to metoclopramide therapy. Br J Oral Surg 1978;15:278–80.
13. Ibrahim ZY, Brooks EF. Neuroleptic-induced bilateral temporomandibular joint dislocation. Am J Psychiatry 1996;153:2–3.

14. Patton DW. Recurrent subluxation of the temporo-mandibular joint in psychiatric illness. Br Dent J 1982;153:141–4.

15. Thexton A. A case of Ehlers-Danlos syndrome presenting with recurrent dislocation of the TMJ. Br J Oral Surg 1965;2:190–3.

16. Vora SB, Feinsod R, Annitto W. Temporomandibular joint dislocation mistaken as dystonia. JAMA 1979; 242:2844.

17. Kai S, Kai H, Wakayama E, et al. Clinical symptoms of open lock position of the condyle. Relation to anterior dislocation of the temporomandibular joint. Oral Surg Oral Med Oral Pathol 1992;74:143–8.

18. Baur DA, Jannuzzi JR, Mercan U, et al. Treatment of long term anterior dislocation of the TMJ. Int J Oral Maxillofac Surg 2013;42(8):1030–3.

19. Huang IY, Chen CM, Kao YH, et al. Management of long-standing mandibular dislocation. Int J Oral Maxillofac Surg 2011;40(8):810–4.

20. Undt G. Temporomandibular joint eminectomy for recurrent dislocation. Atlas Oral Maxillofac Surg Clin North Am 2011;19(2):189–206.

21. Schultz LW. A treatment for subluxation of the temporomandibular joint. JAMA 1937;109(13): 1032–5.

22. Refai H. Long-term therapeutic effects of dextrose prolotherapy in patients with hypermobility of the temporomandibular joint: a single-arm study with 1-4 years' follow up. Br J Oral Maxillofac Surg 2017;55(5):465–70.

23. Banks A. A rationale for prolotherapy. J Orthop Med (UK) 1991;13:54.

24. Cömert Kiliç S, Güngörmüş M. Is dextrose prolotherapy superior to placebo for the treatment of temporomandibular joint hypermobility? A randomized clinical trial. Int J Oral Maxillofac Surg 2016;45(7): 813–9.

25. Refai H, Altahhan O, Elsharkawy R. The efficacy of dextrose prolotherapy for temporomandibular joint hypermobility: a preliminary prospective, randomized, double-blind, placebo-controlled clinical trial. J Oral Maxillofac Surg 2011;69(12): 2962–70.

26. Brachmann F. Autologous blood injection for recurrent hypermobility of the temporomandibular joint. Dtsch Zahnarztl Z 1964;15:97–102 [in German]. Quoted by: Machon V, Abramowicz S, Paska J, et al. Autologous blood injection for the treatment of chronic recurrent temporomandibular joint dislocation. J Oral Maxillofac Surg 2009;67:114–9.

27. Daif ET. Autologous blood injection as a new treatment modality for chronic recurrent temporomandibular joint dislocation. Oral Surg Oral Med Oral Pathol Oral Radiol Endod 2010;109:31–6.

28. Hegab AF. Treatment of chronic recurrent dislocation of the temporomandibular joint with injection of autologous blood alone, intermaxillary fixation alone,

or both together: a prospective, randomized, controlled clinical trial. Br J Oral Maxillofac Surg 2013;51:813–7.

29. Varedi P, Bohluli B. Autologous blood injection for treatment of chronic recurrent TMJ dislocation: is it successful? Is it safe enough? A systematic review. Oral Maxillofac Surg 2015;19(3):243–52.

30. Candirli C, Yüce S, Cavus UY, et al. Autologous blood injection to the temporomandibular joint: magnetic resonance imaging findings. Imaging Sci Dent 2012;42:13–8.

31. Hooiveld M, Roosendaal G, Wenting M, et al. Short-term exposure of cartilage to blood results in chondrocyte apoptosis. Am J Pathol 2003;162:943–51.

32. Roosendaal G, TeKoppele JM, Vianen ME, et al. Blood-induced joint damage: a canine in vivo study. Arthritis Rheum 1999;42:1033–9.

33. Roosendaal G, Vianen ME, Marx JJ, et al. Blood-induced joint damage: a human in vitro study. Arthritis Rheum 1999;42:1025–32.

34. Stembirek J, Matalova E, Buchtova M, et al. Investigation of an autologous blood treatment strategy for temporomandibular joint hypermobility in a pig model. Int J Oral Maxillofac Surg 2013;42:369–75.

35. Daelen B, Thorwirth V, Koch A. Treatment of recurrent dislocation of the temporomandibular joint with type A botulinum toxin. Int J Oral Maxillofac Surg 1997;26:458–60.

36. Majid OW. Clinical use of botulinum toxins in oral and maxillofacial surgery. Int J Oral Maxillofac Surg 2010;39(3):197–207.

37. Vázquez Bouso O, Forteza González G, Mommsen J, et al. Neurogenic temporomandibular joint dislocation treated with botulinum toxin: report of 4 cases. Oral Surg Oral Med Oral Pathol Oral Radiol Endod 2010;109(3):e33–7.

38. Ziegler CM, Haag C, Muhling J. Treatment of recurrent temporomandibular joint dislocation with intramuscular botulinum toxin injection. Clin Oral Investig 2003;7:52–5.

39. Martinez-Perez D, Ruiz-Espiga PG. Recurrent temporomandibular joint dislocation treated with botulinum toxin: report of 3 cases. J Oral Maxillofac Surg 2004;62:244–6.

40. Fu K, Chen HM, Sun ZP, et al. Long term efficacy of botulinum toxin type A for the treatment of habitual dislocation of the temporomandibular joint. Br J Oral Maxillofac Surg 2010;48:281–4.

41. Torres DE, McCain JP. Arthroscopic electrothermal capsulorrhaphy for the treatment of recurrent temporomandibular joint dislocation. Int J Oral Maxillofac Surg 2012;41(6):681–9.

42. McCain JP, Hossameldin RH, Glickman AG. Preliminary clinical experience and outcome of the TMJ arthroscopic chemical contracture procedure in TMJ dislocation patients. J Oral Maxillofac Surg 2014;72(9):e16–7.

43. Ybema A, De Bont LG, Spijkervet FK. Arthroscopic cauterization of retrodiscal tissue as a successful minimal invasive therapy in habitual temporomandibular joint luxation. Int J Oral Maxillofac Surg 2013;42(3):376–9.

44. Boudreaux R, Spire E. Plication of the capsular ligament of the temporomandibular joint: a surgical approach to recurrent dislocation or chronic subluxation. J Oral Surg 1968;26:330–3.

45. Hudson HN. Operation for recurrent subluxation of temporomandibular joint. Br Med J 1945;2:354.

46. MacFarlane WI. Recurrent dislocation of the mandible: treatment of seven cases by a simple surgical method. Br J Oral Surg 1977;14:227–9.

47. Mayer L. Recurrent dislocation of the jaw. J Bone Surg 1933;15:22.

48. LeClerc GC, Girard C. Un nouveau procédé de dute é dans le traitement chirurgical de la luxation recidivante de la machoire inferieur. Mem Acad Chir 1943; 69:457–659.

49. Gosserez M, Dautrey J. Osteoplastic bearing for treatment of temporomandibular luxation. Transaction of Second Congress of the International Association of Oral Surgeons, Copenhagen, Munksgaard. Int J Oral Surg 1967;IV:261.

50. Undt G, Kermer C, Piehslinger E, et al. Treatment of recurrent mandibular dislocation, part 1; LeClerc blocking procedure. Int J Oral Maxillofac Surg 1997;26:92–7.

51. Lawler MG. Recurrent dislocation of the mandible: treatment of ten cases by the Dautrey procedure. Br J Oral Surg 1982;20:14.

52. Gadre KS, Kaul D, Ramanojam S, et al. Dautrey's procedure in treatment of recurrent dislocation of the mandible. J Oral Maxillofac Surg 2010;68(8): 2021–4.

53. Iizuka T, Hidaka Y, Murakami K, et al. Chronic recurrent anterior luxation of the mandible: a review of 12 patients treated by the LeClerc procedure. Int J Oral Maxillofac Surg 1988;17:170–2.

54. Srivastava D, Rajadnya M, Chaudhary MK, et al. The Dautrey procedure in recurrent dislocation: a review of 12 cases. Int J Oral Maxillofac Surg 1994;23:229–31.

55. Kobayashi H, Yamazaki T, Okudera H. Correction of recurrent dislocation of the mandible in elderly patients by the Dautrey procedure. Br J Oral Maxillofac Surg 2000;38:54–7.

56. Smith WP. Recurrent dislocation of the temporomandibular joint. A new combined augmentation procedure. Int J Oral Maxillofac Surg 1991;20:98–9.

57. Revington PJD. The Dautrey procedure—a case for reassessment. Br J Oral Maxillofac Surg 1986;24: 217–20.

58. da Costa Ribeiro R, dos Santos BJ, Provenzano N, et al. Dautrey's procedure: an alternative for the treatment of recurrent mandibular dislocation in patients with pneumatization of the articular eminence. Int J Oral Maxillofac Surg 2014;43(4):465–9.

59. Fernandez-Sanroman J. Surgical treatment of recurrent mandibular dislocation by augmentation of the articular eminence with cranial bone. J Oral Maxillofac Surg 1997;55(4):333–8.

60. Medra A, Mahrous A. Glenotemporal osteotomy and bone grafting in the management of chronic recurrent dislocation and hypermobility of the temporomandibular joint. Br J Oral Maxillofac Surg 2008;46:119–22.

61. Costas Lopez A, Monje Gil F, Fernandez Sanroman J, et al. Glenotemporal osteotomy as a definitive treatment for recurrent dislocation of the jaw. J Craniomaxillofac Surg 1996;24:178–83.

62. Sindet-Pedersen S. Intraoral myotomy of the lateral pterygoid muscle for treatment of recurrent dislocation of the mandibular condyle. J Oral Maxillofac Surg 1968;46:445–9.

63. Miller GA, Murphy EJ. External pterygoid myotomy for recurrent mandibular dislocation. Review of the literature and report of a case. Oral Surg Oral Med Oral Pathol 1976;42:705–16.

64. Laskin DM. Myotomy for the management of recurrent and protracted mandibular dislocations. Transactions of the fourth international conference on oral surgery. Amsterdam, May 17–21, 1971. Copenhagen, Munksgaard; 1973. p. 264–8.

Combined or Staged Temporomandibular Joint and Orthognathic Surgery for Patients with Internal Derangement and Dentofacial Deformities

Somi Kim, DMD, MD[a],*, David A. Keith, BDS, DMD[b]

KEYWORDS

- TMJ • Internal derangement • Dentofacial deformity • Orthognathic surgery
- Temporomandibular disorder

KEY POINTS

- Thorough clinical and radiographic examinations are important to diagnose both the stage of the internal derangement and the dentofacial deformity accurately. It is important to differentiate myofascial pain and dysfunction from intra-articular joint problems.
- Depending on the stage of internal derangement, it can be managed symptomatically with nonsurgical treatment, staged separately with operative management, or treated at the same time as the orthognathic surgery.
- Generally, patients with early and intermediate stages of internal derangement can be managed nonoperatively before orthognathic surgery to reduce pain and increase range of motion and allow orthodontic treatment to proceed. Most of these patients experience an improvement in their TMD symptoms once the dentofacial deformities have been treated.
- Intermediate and intermediate/late-stage internal derangement cases that do not respond to nonsurgical management should have arthrocentesis or arthroscopy before orthognathic surgery, if possible. Otherwise it is preferable to do the orthognathic surgery and if the symptoms do not resolve, open joint surgery can be done.
- Patients with late-stage internal derangement and significant degenerative joint disease will generally require total joint replacement surgery at the same time as orthognathic surgery to achieve stable skeletal and occlusal relationships.

INTRODUCTION

Temporomandibular joint disorders (TMDs) often exist at the same time as dentofacial deformities. Some dentofacial deformities may be a result of a TMD, such as idiopathic condylar resorption or severe degenerative joint disease. Alternatively, these 2 conditions may develop independently. Diagnosis of dentofacial deformities is usually straightforward for oral and maxillofacial surgeons (OMFSs), but diagnosis of TMDs is more challenging.

Disclosure: This work was funded in part by a research education grant (S. Kim) from DePuysynthes (USA).
[a] Private practice, Oral Surgery Partners, 38 SW Cutoff, Northborough, MA 01532, USA; [b] Department of Oral and Maxillofacial Surgery, Massachusetts General Hospital, Warren Suite 1201, 55 Fruit Street, Boston, MA 02114, USA
* Corresponding author.
E-mail address: somikim04@gmail.com

Oral Maxillofacial Surg Clin N Am 30 (2018) 351–354
https://doi.org/10.1016/j.coms.2018.04.010
1042-3699/18/© 2018 Elsevier Inc. All rights reserved.

CLINICAL EVALUATION

It is essential to take a good history, including the patient's chief complaint, symptoms, prior orthodontic treatment history, and treatment expectations. **Box 1** shows the pertinent information to be recorded. As these patients are at high risk for obstructive sleep apnea, every orthognathic surgery patient should be screened with the Epworth sleepiness scale and Stop-Bang score questionnaires.

Physical examination is equally important in evaluating the patient. OMFSs have to be proficient at evaluating patients for both orthognathic surgery and temporomandibular joint dysfunction. **Box 2** shows the overall general information that should be obtained from the physical examination.

It is imperative to obtain all information in "natural head position," as these patients may posture their head "unnaturally" given a myofascial component. It is important to have clinical Frankfort horizontal plane (line from tragus to bony infraorbital rim) parallel to the true horizontal plane.[1]

RADIOGRAPHIC EVALUATION

Imaging is a key component in patient evaluation. All orthognathic patients need a full set of radiographs (panoramic, lateral, and anteroposterior cephalometric radiographs). When panoramic radiography shows significant abnormalities, such as degenerative joint changes, cone-beam computed tomography (CT) or medical grade CT are useful tools to further characterize temporomandibular joint (TMJ) bony morphology and the joint space. This will confirm any significant condylar resorption or degenerative joint disease in the TMJ. Also, the oropharyngeal and nasal airway can be evaluated, especially when obstructive sleep apnea is suspected.[2]

For patients with a suspected internal derangement, MRI allows evaluation of disk morphology, mobility, and position, along with any synovitis or effusion in the joint (see Tore A. Larheim and colleagues' article, "The Role of Imaging in the Diagnosis of Temporomandibular Joint Pathology," in this issue). MRI with gadolinium is especially helpful in visualizing and quantifying the amount of synovitis in the TMJ, especially in patients with a history of juvenile idiopathic arthritis.[3]

CEPHALOMETRIC ANALYSIS

Cephalometric analysis is an important step in diagnosing and treatment planning for patients with dentofacial deformities. Patients with a dentofacial deformity and internal derangement often have an increased occlusal plane angle and clockwise

---

Box 1
Pertinent history when evaluating patients with dentofacial deformity and temporomandibular joint disorder (TMD)

Chief Complaint
- Malocclusion
- Esthetic concerns
- Orofacial pain
- Decreased range of motion of jaw
- Functional concerns, such as difficulty chewing and speaking

Dentofacial Deformity–related History
- Prior orthodontic treatment
- Change in occlusion
- Obstructive sleep apnea questionnaire
  - Epworth sleepiness scale questionnaire
  - Stop-Bang questionnaire
- Growth history

TMD-related History
- Symptoms
  - Pain
  - Range of motion
  - Clicking, crepitus
- Pain
  - Quality
  - Severity
  - Location
  - Radiation
  - Duration
  - Timing
  - Exacerbating and relieving factors
- Prior treatment
  - Medication
  - Physical therapy
  - Splint therapy
  - Surgery
- Prior trauma history
- Parafunctional habit (grinding, clenching)
- Joint noise (crepitus/clicking)
- History of locking
- Change in occlusion
- Medical comorbidities, such as inflammatory joint disease, autoimmune or connective tissue disease, and so forth
- Jaw function, such as diet
- Disability

rotation of the maxillomandibular complex. It is relatively common for these patients to have bimaxillary sagittal hypoplasia, an anterior open bite, an increased occlusal plane, and degenerative TMJ changes.

DENTAL MODEL ANALYSIS

Dental models are used to evaluate the initial occlusal relationship and tooth position as well as orthodontic changes. Analyzing them, and discussing the progress with the patient's orthodontist, is crucial in determining when patients are ready for surgical intervention.

DIAGNOSIS

Diagnoses of the Dentofacial Deformity

Once all the information has been gathered, diagnosing the dentofacial deformity and determining its treatment is relatively straightforward and similar to any other orthognathic surgery treatment plan.

Temporomandibular Joint Dysfunction

Diagnosing a temporomandibular disorder can be difficult and treatment planning is often controversial. It is crucial to differentiate between myofascial pain and dysfunction and intra-articular joint problems. Myofascial pain and dysfunction does not require surgical intervention, but adequate treatment is still needed. Wilkes classification[4] and staging criteria for internal derangement of the TMJ is useful in diagnosing intra-articular joint problems. Myofascial pain commonly accompanies internal derangements and this needs to be managed separately.

TREATMENT PLANNING

Once the diagnoses have been made, the OMFS needs to decide whether to treat the 2 conditions separately or together. This depends on the severity of the symptoms and the diagnoses themselves. Patients with stage I or II internal derangement are generally treated with nonoperative modalities while waiting for orthognathic surgery. This includes jaw rest, soft diet, physical therapy, and medical management (nonsteroidal anti-inflammatory drugs, muscle relaxants). Bite appliance therapy is often difficult when the patient is undergoing orthodontic therapy. In those patients who remain symptomatic, the symptoms often improve after surgery.[5] Otherwise, TMJ surgery can then be done.

For patients with Wilkes stage III or IV internal derangement, and also stage II internal derangements with intermittent locking, it is also important to address the internal derangement first during the orthodontic therapy period before orthognathic surgery. Nonoperative management is again recommended as first-line therapy. If the patient's symptoms persist despite such management, arthroscopy is recommended before orthognathic surgery. Studies show that the overall success rate of arthroscopic lysis and lavage is more than 80% in all Wilkes stages II through V.[6]

For patients with Wilkes stage III or IV who do not have an improvement in their symptoms with arthroscopy, the internal derangement can be managed at the time of orthognathic surgery. Wolford and Dhameja[7] have described simultaneous disk repositioning with a Mitek anchor and orthognathic surgery. They reported good results in patients with anterior disk displacement and little or no previous surgery (0–1 surgery) and less than 4 years since the onset of TMD symptoms.[7] However, we do not recommend routinely doing disk repositioning surgery concurrent with orthognathic surgery. It is our preference to observe patients' symptoms after orthognathic surgery and perform open TMJ surgery, if needed, as a separate procedure. The rationale for delaying the TMJ surgery is that patients' symptoms often improve after orthognathic surgery alone.[5] Also, hypomobility after TMJ surgery is a concern. Patients need active stretching exercises after TMJ surgery and concurrent orthognathic surgery often makes it more difficult for patients to resume active physical therapy.

Once there is a significant degenerative joint disease (Wilkes stage V), the TMJs are not stable enough to withstand orthognathic surgery and the degenerative process may continue. Thus, total joint replacement and reconstruction becomes necessary. These patients are different from the previously discussed patients with Wilkes stage I to IV, as they clearly need TMJ surgery due to the degree of destruction. Reconstruction of the TMJ can be done with an autologous costochondral graft or with alloplastic total joint replacement.[8–12]

SUMMARY

Patients with Wilkes stage I and II types of internal derangement, are generally treated nonsurgically during the orthodontic period preceding orthognathic surgery. Most of these patients remain asymptomatic after correction of the dentofacial deformity. Patients with Wilkes stage III and IV internal derangement who do not respond to nonsurgical therapy should have arthrocentesis or arthroscopy before their orthognathic surgery. If this does not resolve the symptoms, they should have the orthognathic surgery and then open joint surgery if the symptoms continue. Patients with late-stage internal derangement will generally require total joint replacement at the time of orthognathic surgery to achieve stable skeletal and occlusal relationships.

REFERENCES

1. Zebeib AM, Naini FB. Variability of the inclination of anatomic horizontal reference planes of the craniofacial complex in relation to the true horizontal line in orthognathic patients. Am J Orthod Dentofacial Orthop 2014;146:740–7.

2. Abramson ZR, Susarla S, Kaban L, et al. Three-dimensional computed tomographic analysis of airway anatomy. J Oral Maxillofac Surg 2010;68(2): 363–71.

3. Resnick CM, Dang R, Henderson LA, et al. Frequency and morbidity of temporomandibular joint involvement in adult patients with a history of juvenile idiopathic arthritis. J Oral Maxillofac Surg 2017;75:1191–200.

4. Wilkes CH. Internal derangements of the temporomandibular joint. Arch Otolaryngol Head Neck Surg 1989;115:469–77.

5. Al-Moraissi EA, Wolford LM, Perez D, et al. Does orthognathic surgery cause or cure temporomandibular disorders? A systematic review and meta-analysis. J Oral Maxillofac Surg 2017;75: 1835–47.

6. Smolka W, Yanai C, Smolka K, et al. Efficiency of arthroscopic lysis and lavage for internal derangement of the temporomandibular joint correlated with Wilkes classification. Oral Surg Oral Med Oral Pathol Oral Radiol Endod 2008;106:317–23.

7. Wolford LM, Dhameja A. Planning for combined TMJ arthroplasty and orthognathic surgery. Atlas Oral Maxillofac Surg Clin North Am 2011;19:243–70.

8. Giannakopoulos HE, Sinn DP, Quinn PD. Biomet microfixation temporomandibular joint replacement system: a 3-year follow up study of patients treated during 1995 to 2005. J Oral Maxillofac Surg 2012;70: 787–94.

9. Mercuri LG, Wolford LM, Sanders B, et al. Long-term follow-up of the CAD/CAM patient fitted total temporomandibular joint reconstruction system. J Oral Maxillofac Surg 2002;60:1440–8.

10. Mercuri LG, Edibam NR, Giobbie-Hurder A. Fourteen-year follow-up of a patient-fitted total temporomandibular joint reconstruction system. J Oral Maxillofac Surg 2007;65:1140–8.

11. Zou L, He D, Ellis E. A comparison of clinical follow-up of different total temporomandibular joint replacement prostheses: a systematic review and meta-analysis. J Oral Maxillofac Surg 2018;76(2): 294–303.

12. Mercuri LG. Alloplastic temporomandibular joint replacement: rationale for the use of custom devices. Int J Oral Maxillofac Surg 2012;41:1033–40.

Surgical Management of Idiopathic Condylar Resorption
Orthognathic Surgery Versus Temporomandibular Total Joint Replacement

Radhika Chigurupati, DMD, MS, Pushkar Mehra, BDS, DMD*

KEYWORDS

- Idiopathic condylar resorption • Costochondral graft • Orthognathic surgery
- Total joint replacement

KEY POINTS

- Idiopathic condylar resorption (ICR) classically affects young women with a Class II malocclusion and high mandibular plane angle.
- It results in progressive reduction in condylar size, and alteration of condylar contour and shape; sometimes accompanied by symptoms of pain and functional limitations.
- The resulting facial deformity can cause disability due to the open bite malocclusion, unaesthetic profile, and difficulty with mastication and speech.
- Orthognathic surgery alone for ICR should not be done until clinical examination and diagnostic investigation have established that the active changes in the condyles have stopped.
- Temporomandibular joint replacement with alloplastic prosthesis alone, or combined with orthognathic surgery, offers a definitive treatment option for patients with final-stage ICR or persistent condylar activity. It eliminates the morbidity of a second surgical site, and the risk of undergrowth or overgrowth that can occur with a costochondral graft.

INTRODUCTION

Idiopathic condylar resorption (ICR) is an acquired disorder of the temporomandibular joint (TMJ) classically affecting young women between 15 and 40 years of age, which causes progressive reduction of condylar volume leading to alteration of contour and shape. It can be asymptomatic or present with symptoms of joint pain and dysfunction. Occasionally, it can be unilateral and affect men.[1–5] Although some patients have only minimal functional limitations, the resulting changes in facial appearance and the open bite malocclusion often lead to difficulty with chewing and speech, as well as airway and breathing disorders in severe cases.

The correction of the facial skeletal deformity and malocclusion in patients with ICR can be challenging because of the unpredictable duration of the condition and the variable extent of

Disclosure: The authors have nothing to disclose.
Department of Oral and Maxillofacial Surgery, Boston University, Henry M. Goldman School of Dental Medicine, 100 East Newton Street, Suite G-407, Boston, MA 02118, USA
* Corresponding author.
E-mail address: pmehra@bu.edu

Oral Maxillofacial Surg Clin N Am 30 (2018) 355–367
https://doi.org/10.1016/j.coms.2018.05.004
1042-3699/18/

the condylar changes. Operative intervention has to be selected and timed appropriately, after clinical examination and diagnostic investigations have collectively established that condylar activity has either ceased spontaneously or is to be arrested by the surgical procedure.[6] The ultimate goal of treatment for patients with ICR is to achieve a stable occlusion without relapse, adequate jaw function, and balanced facial proportions.

The surgical treatment of ICR remains controversial and there are only a few case series and/or meta-analyses to date discussing the various options. Generally speaking, the treatment options include some form of orthognathic surgery with or without TMJ surgery.[7–14] In this article, we discuss the controversies in the management of ICR along with the pros and cons of 2 surgical options: orthognathic surgery alone or orthognathic surgery and total joint replacement. The etiology of ICR, its clinical presentation and diagnosis, and the investigations required before surgical treatment also are briefly reviewed.

HISTORY AND ETIOLOGY

Reports of ICR were published in 1961 by Burke,[15] in 1977 by Rabey[16] and Norman,[17] and by Lanigan and colleagues[18] as a case report of a patient with a collagen disorder in 1979. Since the initial description, several others have reported on this condition, often diagnosed after unexplained relapse after orthognathic surgery.[18–22] The treatment of ICR has evolved in the past 2 decades with the advent of alloplastic reconstruction of the TMJ.[23–25] The exact cause or stimulus that initiates or propagates the process is unknown, although many contributing factors have been suggested. It has been reported to occur after increased mechanical loading of the TMJ following orthodontic treatment, orthognathic surgery, trauma, internal derangement, occlusal therapy, or parafunctional habits.[2,3,19,26–30] Wolford and Cardenas[29] have suggested that the condylar resorption in patients with ICR is mediated by morphologic and secretory changes in the hypertrophic bilaminar zone of the TMJ disk. Others have argued that avascular necrosis might play a role in the pathogenesis of ICR.[31] Hormonal mediation based on the presence of estrogen receptors in the human TMJ and the influence of estrogen and prolactin on bone response have also been proposed as etiologies.[32–35] In most cases, however, no clear identifiable cause is evident and hence the condition is generally referred to as ICR.

EPIDEMIOLOGY AND CLINICAL PRESENTATION

ICR, also sometimes referred to as progressive condylar resorption or adult ICR in the literature, occurs infrequently, with a reported prevalence of 1:5000 among individuals presenting for orthodontic treatment.[30] Condylar resorption as a complication among all individuals undergoing orthognathic surgery is reported to occur in the range of 2% to 5%, and, within the subset of patients with Class II malocclusion with steep mandibular plane angles, its incidence is even higher (19%–31%).[30] There is a high female predilection for this condition and a peak incidence between the ages of 15 to 35 years (average age: 20.5 years), and a male-to-female ratio of 1:9. The early symptoms and signs of condylar resorption are subtle; they may or may not be present before orthodontic treatment or orthognathic surgery, but become more apparent after treatment. Resorption is usually slow, approximately 1.0 to 1.5 mm per year, so it initially may be difficult to identify clinically, especially if the orthodontist is compensating for the ongoing skeletal changes with counteracting dental movement(s). As the condylar resorption progresses, individuals classically present with a gradually retruding chin, anterior open bite, loss of posterior facial height, clockwise rotation of the mandible, and development of retrognathia with or without associated symptoms of TMJ pain and functional limitations. It is not uncommon to find that patients with ICR give a history of being managed by multiple providers in the medical and dental specialties. **Fig. 1** demonstrates the typical clinical and radiographic presentation of a patient with early ICR.

RISK FACTORS FOR CONDYLAR RESORPTION

The risk factors can be broadly classified into 2 categories: patient-related or surgery-related (**Box 1**). Patient risk factors include age, gender, physiology, medications, systemic disorders, mandibular anatomy, bone density, and dental occlusion. Among the orthognathic surgery population, young women with a Class II malocclusion, mandibular retrognathism with an anterior open bite, high or wide mandibular plane angles, a low posterior-to-anterior facial height ratio, and a slender posteriorly inclined condylar neck are at known to be at high risk for ICR.[22,36,37] Condyles with preexisting radiological signs of osteoarthritis also may be at higher risk for progressive resorption.[36] O'Ryan and Epker[38] evaluated the morphologic changes in the condyle and studied the

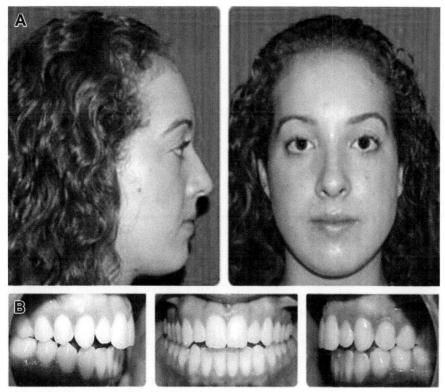

Fig. 1. (*A*) Clinical frontal and profile view of a patient with ICR. Note Class II skeletal profile with a retrusive chin point. (*B*) Intraoral views of the same patient's occlusion. The patient started to develop a slowly worsening open bite during active orthodontic treatment.

radiographic features in individuals presenting for orthognathic surgery. They found less dense and less discreetly oriented trabeculae in patients with a high mandibular plane angle compared with patients with a low mandibular plane angle when they assessed bone density and orientation of the trabeculae of the condyles.[38] Also noted was that patients with a steep mandibular plane tended to have smaller condyles compared with those with a flat mandibular plane. The ratio of cortical to cancellous bone in teenagers and adolescents is less compared with adults, and this may be one of the reasons for increased susceptibility to condylar resorption and remodeling in young teenagers.[39] Orthodontists and oral and maxillofacial surgeons treating individuals for correction of a malocclusion must recognize the various demographic features and mandibular anatomic findings and identify high-risk patients before treatment.

Surgical risk factors include the magnitude and direction of mandibular movement, type of surgical fixation, and length of postoperative maxillomandibular fixation (MMF). A few investigators have evaluated changes in the bone associated with abnormal joint loading after surgery. They have documented that the condyles may be torqued when rigid fixation is used to secure the proximal and distal segments, in particular during sagittal split osteotomy. Excessive pressure on the lateral or medial pole of the condyle can lead to condylar resorption and subsequent clinical relapse after orthognathic surgery.[2,3,21] Hwang and colleagues[40] noted condylar resorption on the superior and antero-superior aspects of the condylar head when there is posterior displacement of the condyle and counterclockwise rotation of the distal and proximal segments in patients undergoing mandibular osteotomies. Condylar resorption after orthognathic surgery was greater in susceptible patients who undergo mandibular advancements of 10 mm or greater. It was also shown to be greater in the group with intraosseous wire fixation and postoperative MMF than in cases with rigid internal fixation without MMF.[22] Wolford and colleagues[41] reported significant worsening of the TMJ dysfunction after orthognathic surgery in patients with documented clinical and imaging (MRI scan) evidence of preoperative TMJ internal derangement. Six (24%) of their 25 patients developed condylar resorption with a Class II malocclusion and an open bite postsurgically.

DIAGNOSTIC CONSIDERATIONS

When condylar resorption is suspected based on changes in the occlusion and unexplained relapse after orthodontic treatment or orthognathic surgery, or TMJ dysfunction, advanced imaging and hematologic investigations are necessary to establish the diagnosis. In advanced cases, a panoramic radiograph is a useful screening tool to assess reduction in volume, changes in shape, and the articular surface of the condyle and loss of mandibular ramus height. In individuals with a high suspicion of ICR, cone beam computed tomography provides valuable information regarding the size, shape, quality, articular surfaces, and relationship of the osseous components of the TMJ.[22,42,43] TMJs of adolescents affected by ICR show disappearance of the cortical layer, resorption and irregularity of the condylar surface, as well as subcortical cyst formation.[44] These degenerative bony alterations are frequently accompanied by pain.[45]

To assess quantitative or qualitative interval changes in the size and shape of the condyle, it is important to image the TMJ properly with an axially corrected technique to acquire sectional images perpendicular and parallel to the mediolateral long axis of the condyles. Visualization of the soft tissues, that is, the articular disc and periarticular tissues, and assessment of the cortical and marrow changes in the condyle, requires MRI.[46] More recently, specific TMJ MRI findings for synovial diseases and ICR have been published, and it is expected that as this technology and its interpretation improve, MRI examination will likely play an important role in diagnosis and management of patients with TMJ condylar resorption. Condylar activity also can be assessed by skeletal scintigraphy (quantifiable TC 99 scans with single-photon emission computed tomography and/or planar imaging), which helps to determine whether the condylar resorption is active, thus guiding treatment decisions. Performing a radioisotope study as part of the diagnosis of ICR is valuable, but it cannot differentiate condylar activity due to ICR from other inflammatory and hyperactivity conditions. The interpretation of quantitative measurements of the radioisotope uptake also may vary.[47–49]

SURGICAL MANAGEMENT OF PATIENTS WITH IDIOPATHIC CONDYLAR RESORPTION

The ideal surgical treatment of ICR remains controversial. One of most challenging aspects of treatment is the difficulty in assessing whether condylar resorption is active. Condylar resorption continues in most individuals for a variable period and its duration is unpredictable. Papadaki and colleagues[5] reported in 2007 that condylar resorption can become inactive after 1 to 5 years, but the resorptive process may be reactivated. Therefore, it is important to distinguish between active and inactive condylar resorption. They also stated that the resorptive process rarely continues beyond 40 years of age, although this finding has not been confirmed by other researchers.

In a review of the existing literature, the most common surgical treatment options for management of the deformity resulting from ICR are orthognathic surgery alone[7,13,50,51] or combined TMJ and orthognathic surgery[11,23,52,53] (**Box 2**). The specific type of TMJ procedure reported varies in different articles. A few clinicians have even advocated the use of distraction osteogenesis, although it is not popular.[54] Irrespective of the type of surgical management, it is essential to first exclude known local and systemic causes of TMJ condylar resorption (eg, autoimmune/connective tissue diseases, hormonal deficiencies, endocrine disturbances, trauma, prior TMJ surgery, TMJ pathology) by serial clinical

Box 2
Surgical treatment options for dentofacial deformity due to idiopathic condylar resorption

1. Orthognathic surgery alone
2. Orthognathic surgery with TMJ surgery (staged or concomitant)
   a. Orthognathic surgery with disk repositioning or stabilization
   b. Orthognathic surgery with TMJ replacement (autogenous/alloplastic)

prosthesis (25/210) was the treatment of choice in a third (33%) of the patients. Nonsurgical management of symptoms, or orthodontic treatment, was performed in 21 (10%) of 210 patients. They reported that the results of treatment were variable for the orthognathic surgery group, with postoperative stability ranging from 57% to 100%; in contrast, those patients who had total joint reconstruction had 95% to 100% postoperative stability with a follow-up period ranging between 3 months and 11 years. They proposed an algorithm based on condylar activity and the surgeon's ability to salvage the disk and mandibular condyle.

examinations, appropriate diagnostic imaging, laboratory investigations, and consultation with an experienced rheumatologist.

In a recent systematic review, Sansare and colleagues[14] reported on the radiologic findings and treatment outcomes of patients treated for ICR with different management approaches. **Table 1** summarizes their findings. Zuleima and colleagues[13] also conducted a review on management of the dentofacial deformity caused by condylar resorption. Their search resulted in 21 articles with a total of 210 cases of ICR treated between 1991 and 2012. Orthognathic surgery alone was the most common treatment performed in 72 (34%) of 210 patients; orthognathic surgery with concomitant TMJ surgery was performed in 46 (21%) of 210 patients and condylectomy and TMJ reconstruction with a costochondral graft (36/210) or alloplastic TMJ

THE CASE FOR ORTHOGNATHIC SURGERY ALONE FOR MANAGEMENT OF IDIOPATHIC CONDYLAR RESORPTION

The rationale for orthognathic surgery alone in the management of the dentofacial deformity that ensues from ICR is based on the assumption that the condylar resorption is triggered by some biomechanical or physiologic stimulus that is transient. As the instigating stimulus ceases, the condyles should become quiescent, and the malocclusion and skeletal deformity should be amenable for correction with orthognathic surgery alone by taking certain factors into consideration (**Box 3**). The surgeon must assess the severity of dentofacial deformity to determine if it can be corrected to achieve the desired facial change and occlusion, assess the degree/quantity of condylar resorption, determine

Table 1
Outcomes of idiopathic condylar resorption treatment

Author and Year	Management Approach (n)	Relapse (%)	Follow-up Period, mo
Arnett & Tamborello,[1] 1990	Orthognathic surgery (6)	5 (83.3)	1–39
Crawford et al,[7] 1994	Orthognathic surgery (6)	5 (71.4)	12–68
Merkx & van Damme,[28] 1994	Orthognathic surgery (4)	4 (100)	27
	Occlusal splint and orthodontic treatment (4)	0 (0)	
Wolford & Cardenas,[29] 1995, 1999	Orthognathic + TMJ Disk repositioning (12)	0 (0)	18–68
Hoppenreijs et al,[8] 1999	Splint, orthodontics (13)	0 (0)	24
	Orthognathic surgery (13)	6 (46.1)	
Teitelbaum et al,[12] 2007	Orthognathic surgery (10)	0 (0)	12
Mercuri,[9] 2007	Alloplastic TMJ (5)	0 (0)	>12
Troulis et al,[11] 2008	Autogenous TMJ (15)	0 (0)	>12

Adapted from Sansare K, Raghav M, Mallya SM, et al. Management-related outcomes and radiographic findings of idiopathic condylar resorption: a systematic review. Int J Oral Maxillofac Surg 2015;44(2):213; with permission.

the presence or absence TMJ dysfunction, and confirm the absence of condylar activity for a period at least 12 months (and preferably up to 24 months, because the resorption in most cases is of small magnitude and difficult to detect: approximately 1.0–1.5 mm/y) by serial clinical monitoring and imaging studies. Other anatomic findings that may dictate the surgeon's decision toward performing orthognathic surgery alone include a stable posterior facial height to anterior facial height ratio and no change in ramus length, chin position, or occlusion (overjet) at 2 time points at least 6 to 12 months apart. The presence of TMJ dysfunction and a displaced intra-articular disk, and decreased bone mineral density using a dual-energy X-ray absorptiometry scan, also have been reported as factors that may adversely affect the outcome of orthognathic surgery in patients with ICR.[52] Use of an orthotic appliance and perioperative medical therapy have the potential to reduce the risk of condylar resorption when orthognathic surgery is performed in patients with ICR patients.[51] Patients with complete resorption of the condylar head and/or the posterior facial height is <35 mm may not always be good candidates for orthognathic surgery. Huang and colleagues[10] reported that condylectomy and replacement with a costochondral graft was more stable than orthognathic surgery alone in this subgroup, although it was difficult to predict preoperatively who would benefit most from this treatment modality. Based on their clinical experience, they postulated that the end point of ICR occurs when the condyle is resorbed to the sigmoid notch. When patients have a residual condylar mass and are treated by orthognathic surgery, further condylar resorption can always occur, resulting in relapse.

PRECAUTIONS IF ORTHOGNATHIC SURGERY ALONE IS USED IN PATIENTS WITH IDIOPATHIC CONDYLAR RESORPTION

When orthognathic surgery alone is to be performed for correction of open bite deformities in patients with ICR, the surgeon should consider correction of the malocclusion with maxillary surgery only, if possible (**Fig. 2**). Mandibular surgery carries the risk of reinitiation of resorption even in stable cases due to factors described later in this article. If mandibular surgery is necessary, movements of large magnitude that will increase the biomechanical strain on the TMJ and surrounding muscles should be avoided. One may want to consider an augmentation procedure, such as a genioplasty, along with the mandibular advancement, rather than a large mandibular advancement by itself. Conservative TMJ management principles always should be included in the treatment while a more definitive treatment plan is being formulated. The objective of such conservative therapy is to decrease loading of the joint and minimize pain and dysfunction with orthotic appliances, orthodontics, and pharmaceutical therapy. It is important to ensure that condylar activity is arrested and symptoms of TMJ dysfunction are absent or decreased before orthognathic surgery. This could occur spontaneously (ie, the condylar resorption becomes quiescent), or be achieved with the previously mentioned conservative measures and target-directed pharmaceutical therapy.[51]

WHY NOT TO PERFORM ORTHOGNATHIC SURGERY ALONE?

Most published studies have demonstrated less than ideal outcomes, with a high rate of relapse, when orthognathic surgery alone is used for treating ICR.[14] Crawford and colleagues[7] found that 5 of their 7 patients with ICR had reactivation of condylar resorption after orthognathic surgery. It has also been reported that revision osteotomy may be required in 50% of patients with ICR due to poor esthetics and occlusal instability after orthognathic surgery procedures.[28] Huang and colleagues[10] reported less than optimal results with orthognathic surgery alone in patients with ICR even though there was inactive condylar resorption. Four (24%) of the 18 patients had skeletal relapse, whereas 4 others had stable occlusal results but developed adverse temporomandibular disorder (TMD) symptoms after surgery. However, the proponents of orthognathic surgery continue to contend that it is less invasive than TMJ surgery

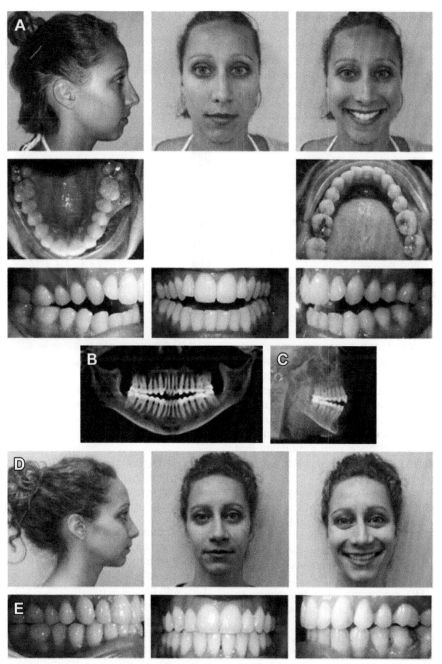

Fig. 2. (*A*) Preoperative extraoral and intraoral views of a 26-year old female patient with history of ICR. She was monitored by her orthodontist and surgeon for 8 years and the ICR was deemed stable with no active resorption for the last 5+ years. (*B*) Preoperative panoramic radiograph reconstruction demonstrating advanced resorption of condyles. (*C*) Preoperative cephalometric radiograph reconstruction demonstrating Class II skeletal relationship with anterior open bite malocclusion. Note steep mandibular and occlusal planes with decreased posterior vertical facial height. (*D*) Postoperative frontal and profile views of the same patient 2+ years after maxillary Le Fort 1 osteotomy only. Note that despite closure of the open bite deformity, the overall facial profile remains convex because the mandible was not surgically advanced. (*E*) Patient's occlusion at the 2+ year postoperative interval. The occlusion has remained stable because condylar resorption was not reinitiated after maxillary surgery.

and should at least be considered for cases in which the resorption has been arrested. Because mandibular orthognathic surgery alone in patients with ICR has high relapse rates due to the persistence or reactivation of the disease, historically speaking, maxillary surgery has often been labeled as "safe to perform" and shown to be effective in closing open bite cases in patients with inactive/stable condyles. However, the primary problem in patients with ICR is the mandible and not the maxilla! Some clinicians also have recommended that delaying orthognathic surgery for a few years after the condition "burns out" may increase the stability of traditional orthognathic surgery. However, there is no objective scientific evidence to support that this delay in treatment will increase long-term predictability and success.

In summary, there are multiple disadvantages to the "orthognathic surgery alone" approach:

1. ICR is a poorly understood process that can undergo periods of reactivation and remission. What one sees presurgery may not be the case postsurgery! An inactive case can become active later in the patient's lifetime, which would render the orthognathic operation a failure and likely require a repeated operation, including TMJ surgery. These patients are usually young, and they should be treated once with a modality that is potentially curative to give them the best quality of life.
2. Although maxillary orthognathic surgery can be used to close an open bite by selective posterior impaction, this procedure, and the associated jaw repositioning movement, does not correct the mandibular retrognathism, which is the primary problem in patients with ICR. Additionally, improvement in the airway, reduction of TMD symptoms, and the ability to restore optimal facial balance and esthetics is limited with this approach.[4,22]
3. Advancing the lower jaw physically lengthens the Class III lever arm of the mandible, which is known to increase loading on the TMJ. Thus, any mandibular advancement surgery increases the risk of postsurgical condylar remodeling and possibly renewed resorption and relapse (**Fig. 3**).
4. With less than ideal anatomic TMJs and preexisting joint "instability," ICR development or reinitiation, worsening of temporomandibular dysfunction, and surgical relapse is to be expected postsurgically in a significant percentage of patients who are treated with orthognathic surgery alone (**Fig. 4**).

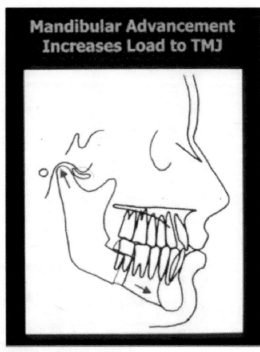

Fig. 3. Schematic representation of the mandible and TMJ working together as a Class III lever. As the mandible is advanced anteriorly, the length of the lever arm increases, thereby increasing TMJ loading during function.

WHY SHOULD ONE PERFORM ALLOPLASTIC TEMPOROMANDIBULAR JOINT RECONSTRUCTION IN PATIENTS WITH IDIOPATHIC CONDYLAR RESORPTION?

TMJ reconstruction in patients with condylar resorption has traditionally been performed using costochondral grafts,[10,11] and, more recently, using prosthetic TMJ total joint replacement (TJR) with favorable results.[53,55–60] Costochondral grafts undergo remodeling and resorption, which can lead to postsurgical occlusion changes. They are prone to ankylosis and do not give the stability, esthetics or quality of jaw function that a properly implanted, prosthetic custom-made, alloplastic prosthetic device delivers (**Fig. 5**). Reasons to use an alloplastic prosthesis as the first choice in the surgical treatment of patients with ICR include the following[53,55–58]:

1. It eliminates the morbidity of a second surgical site.
2. There is no postsurgical remodeling so the mandibular position remains stable.
3. The longevity of the prostheses is no longer questionable because there are reports of more than 20 years of follow-up.[59,60]

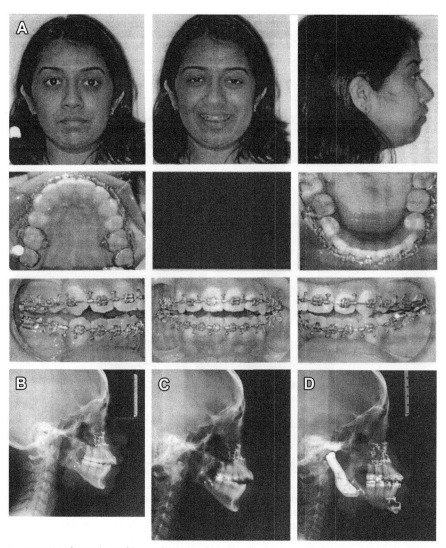

Fig. 4. (*A*) Preoperative frontal, profile, and intraoral views of a 22-year-old female patient before orthognathic surgery. (*B*) Six-month postoperative cephalometric radiograph showing development of a Class II, open bite malocclusion. The occlusion immediately after orthognathic surgery (Le Fort I and bilateral sagittal split osteotomies) was Class I, but the patient started to develop progressive mandibular retrusion with severe, worsening TMJ pain approximately 3 months after surgery. (*C*) Cephalometric radiograph at the 15-month postoperative interval after orthognathic surgery. Note that the open bite has worsened with further mandibular retrusion due to continued condylar resorption. (*D*) Cephalometric radiograph after corrective, revision surgery. This patient underwent bilateral TMJ total joint alloplastic replacement, mandibular counterclockwise advancement, and ramus lengthening, Le Fort I osteotomy, and genioplasty.

4. TMJ alloplastic prostheses lack growth potential, but growth is not required in patients with ICR who have achieved skeletal maturity.
5. These prostheses do not have the problem of unpredictable undergrowth or overgrowth that is frequently seen with costochondral grafts.
6. Most patients with ICR benefit from mandibular advancement and, specifically, lengthening of the posterior facial height (see **Fig. 5**G). This is achieved optimally by counterclockwise rotation of maxillomandibular complex, which

improves the esthetic outcome by restoring the lost posterior facial height and facilitating greater mandibular advancement at Point B and pogonion (see **Fig. 5**H).[55] However, as this type of surgical movement increases TMJ loading biomechanically, it has often been described as a predisposing factor for causing worsening of TMDs and a factor for relapse after orthognathic surgery, especially after autogenous reconstruction.[58] On the other hand, using a prosthetic joint replacement

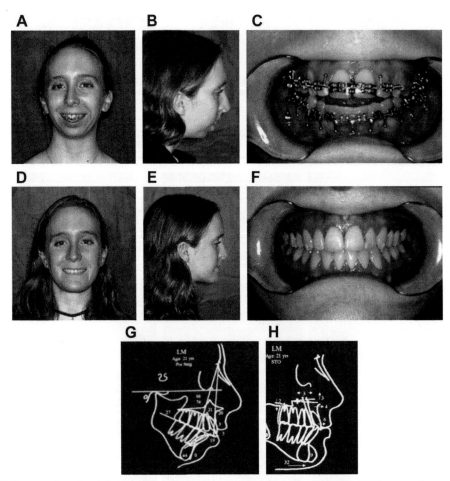

Fig. 5. (*A*) Preoperative frontal view of a 21-year-old woman with advanced ICR. (*B*) Preoperative profile view showing severe mandibular retrusion and Class II skeletal deformity. Such patients with advanced resorption often have compensatory vertical maxillary excess if the disorder manifests during growing years. They also have a predisposition to obstructive sleep apnea development due to the retruded mandibular position and inferior displacement of the hyoid bone. (*C*) Preoperative occlusion (Class II, open bite). (*D*) Postoperative frontal view 4 years after bilateral TMJ TJR, mandibular advancement, Le Fort I osteotomy, and chin augmentation. (See legend for [*H*] for surgical details). (*E*) Postoperative profile view. (*F*) Postoperative occlusion 4 years after concomitant TMJ and orthognathic surgery. (*G*) Preoperative cephalometric measurements demonstrating Class II skeletal relationship and loss of posterior facial height in an ICR patient. Note steep mandibular and occlusal planes. (*H*) The patient was treated with restoration of the posterior facial height by mandibular ramus lengthening with the patient-fitted TMJ prostheses. The occlusal and mandibular planes were normalized by counterclockwise rotation of the maxillomandibular complex. The mandible was advanced anteriorly by 23 mm at Point B and a 9-mm chin implant placed for additional cosmetic benefit. A Le Fort I osteotomy with posterior downgrafting was performed to achieve a normal Class I occlusion and correction of the vertical maxillary excess. (*Courtesy of [A–F]* Dr Larry M. Wolford, Dallas, TX.)

along with orthognathic surgery to achieve this movement has been repeatedly shown to be extremely stable because the prosthesis does not remodel or resorb.

SUMMARY

Clinicians treating young patients for correction of dentofacial deformities should recognize clinical signs, such as a retruded mandible, a short ramus height, and a Class II open bite malocclusion with or without TMD, as high-risk factors for ICR. Such patients should be appropriately informed of the risk of relapse and possible need for further treatment. Both orthognathic surgery and TJR are acceptable surgical treatment options for management of the deformity that ensues from ICR. Proper patient selection for each treatment option is important. Although orthognathic surgery alone is contraindicated in the actively resorbing stage, it could be potentially used in stable cases with certain precautions and considerations. However, long-term occlusal stability cannot be guaranteed with this approach. The evidence-based literature suggests that alloplastic joint replacement along with orthognathic surgery, although more invasive, may be the preferred approach for most patients, especially when there is complete loss of the condyle. The ultimate goal of treatment, whichever method is used, is to ensure that IMJ condylar resorption has ceased or is surgically arrested, that a stable occlusion with a functional jaw joint is achieved, and that facial esthetics are improved.

REFERENCES

1. Arnett GW. Progressive class II development: female idiopathic condylar resorption. Oral Maxillofac Surg Clin North Am 1990;2:699–716.
2. Arnett GW, Milam SB, Gottesman L. Progressive mandibular retrusion–idiopathic condylar resorption. Part I. Am J Orthod Dentofacial Orthop 1996;110(1): 8–15.
3. Arnett GW, Milam SB, Gottesman L. Progressive mandibular retrusion-idiopathic condylar resorption. Part II. Am J Orthod Dentofacial Orthop 1996; 110(2):117–27.
4. Arnett GW, Tamborello JA. TMJ dysfunction from transorally placed lag screws: fact or fiction? J Oral Maxillofac Surg 1988;46(7):625.
5. Papadaki ME, Tayebaty F, Kaban LB, et al. Condylar resorption. Oral Maxillofac Surg Clin North Am 2007; 19(2):223–34, vii.
6. Laskin DM, Hylander WL, editors. Temporomandibular joint disorders. Hanover Park (IL): Quintessence; 2006.
7. Crawford JG, Stoelinga PJ, Blijdorp PA, et al. Stability after reoperation for progressive condylar resorption after orthognathic surgery: report of seven cases. J Oral Maxillofac Surg 1994;52(5):460–6.
8. Hoppenreijs TJ, Stoelinga PJ, Grace KL, et al. Long-term evaluation of patients with progressive condylar resorption following orthognathic surgery. Int J Oral Maxillofac Surg 1999;28(6):411–8.
9. Mercuri LG. A rationale for total alloplastic temporomandibular joint reconstruction in the management of idiopathic/progressive condylar resorption. J Oral Maxillofac Surg 2007;65(8):1600–9.
10. Huang YL, Pogrel MA, Kaban LB. Diagnosis and management of condylar resorption. J Oral Maxillofac Surg 1997;55(2):114–9 [discussion: 119–20].
11. Troulis MJ, Tayebaty FT, Papadaki M, et al. Condylectomy and costochondral graft reconstruction for treatment of active idiopathic condylar resorption. J Oral Maxillofac Surg 2008;66(1):65–72.
12. Wolford LM, Goncalves JR. Condylar resorption of the temporomandibular joint: how do we treat it? Oral Maxillofac Surg Clin North Am 2015; 27(1):47–67.
13. Zuleima C, Breton P, Bouletreau P. Management of dentoskeletal deformity due to condylar resorption: literature review. Oral Surg Oral Med Oral Pathol Oral Radiol 2016;121(2):126–32.
14. Sansare KM, Raghav M, Mallya SM, et al. Management-related outcomes and radiographic findings of idiopathic condylar resorption: a systematic review. Int J Oral Maxillofac Surg 2015; 44(2):209–16.
15. Burke PH. A case of acquired unilateral mandibular condylar hypoplasia. Proc R Soc Med 1961; 54:507–10.
16. Rabey GP. Bilateral mandibular condylysis—a morphanalytic diagnosis. Br J Oral Surg 1977;15(2): 121–34.
17. Norman JE. Surgical diseases of the mandible. The principles of diagnosis and treatment. Aust Dent J 1977;22(2):132–8.
18. Lanigan DT, Myall RW, West RA, et al. Condylysis in a patient with a mixed collagen vascular disease. Oral Surg Oral Med Oral Pathol 1979;48(3):198–204.
19. Bouwman JP, Kerstens HC, Tuinzing DB. Condylar resorption in orthognathic surgery. The role of intermaxillary fixation. Oral Surg Oral Med Oral Pathol 1994;78(2):138–41.
20. De Clercq CA, Neyt LF, Mommaerts MY, et al. Condylar resorption in orthognathic surgery: a retrospective study. Int J Adult Orthodon Orthognath Surg 1994;9(3):233–40.
21. Cutbirth M, Van Sickels JE, Thrash WJ. Condylar resorption after bicortical screw fixation of mandibular advancement. J Oral Maxillofac Surg 1998; 56(2):178–82 [discussion: 183].
22. Hoppenreijs TJ, Freihofer HP, Stoelinga PJ, et al. Condylar remodelling and resorption after Le Fort I and bimaxillary osteotomies in patients with anterior open bite. A clinical and radiological study. Int J Oral Maxillofac Surg 1998;27(2):81–91.
23. Mercuri LG, Ali FA, Woolson R. Outcomes of total alloplastic replacement with periarticular autogenous fat grafting for management of reankylosis of the temporomandibular joint. J Oral Maxillofac Surg 2008;66(9):1794–803.
24. Chung CJ, Choi YJ, Kim IS, et al. Total alloplastic temporomandibular joint reconstruction combined with orthodontic treatment in a patient with idiopathic condylar resorption. Am J Orthod Dentofacial Orthop 2011;140(3):404–17.
25. Movahed R, Wolford LM. Protocol for concomitant temporomandibular joint custom-fitted total joint reconstruction and orthognathic surgery using computer-assisted surgical simulation. Oral Maxillofac Surg Clin North Am 2015;27(1):37–45.
26. Sesenna E, Raffaini M. Bilateral condylar atrophy after combined osteotomy for correction of mandibular

retrusion. A case report. J Maxillofac Surg 1985;
13(6):263–6.

27. Tanaka E, Detamore MS, Mercuri LG. Degenerative
disorders of the temporomandibular joint: etiology,
diagnosis, and treatment. J Dent Res 2008;87(4):
296–307.

28. Merkx MA, Van Damme PA. Condylar resorption
after orthognathic surgery. Evaluation of treatment
in 8 patients. J Craniomaxillofac Surg 1994;22(1):
53–8.

29. Wolford LM, Cardenas L. Idiopathic condylar
resorption: diagnosis, treatment protocol, and
outcomes. Am J Orthod Dentofacial Orthop 1999;
116(6):667–77.

30. Handelman CG. Progressive/idiopathic condylar
resorption: an orthodontic perspective. Semin Orthod 2013;19(2):55–70.

31. Chuong R, Piper MA. Avascular necrosis of the
mandibular condyle-pathogenesis and concepts of
management. Oral Surg Oral Med Oral Pathol
1993;75(4):428–32.

32. Haskin CL, Milam SB, Cameron IL. Pathogenesis of
degenerative joint disease in the human temporomandibular joint. Crit Rev Oral Biol Med 1995;6(3):
248–77.

33. Milam SB, Aufdemorte TB, Sheridan PJ, et al. Sexual
dimorphism in the distribution of estrogen receptors
in the temporomandibular joint complex of the ba-
boon. Oral Surg Oral Med Oral Pathol 1987;64(5):
527–32.

34. Wolford LM. Idiopathic condylar resorption of the
temporomandibular joint in teenage girls (cheer-
leaders syndrome). Proc (Bayl Univ Med Cent)
2001;14(3):246–52.

35. Gunson MJ, Arnett GW. Pathophysiology and pharmacologic control of osseous mandibular condylar
resorption. Response. J Oral Maxillofac Surg 2013;
71(1):4.

36. Kerstens HC, Tuinzing DB, Golding RP, et al.
Condylar atrophy and osteoarthrosis after bimaxillary surgery. Oral Surg Oral Med Oral Pathol 1990;
69(3):274–80.

37. Hwang SJ, Haers PE, Seifert B, et al. Non-surgi-
cal risk factors for condylar resorption after
orthognathic surgery. J Craniomaxillofac Surg
2004;32(2):103–11.

38. O'Ryan F, Epker BN. Temporomandibular joint function and morphology: observations on the spectra of
normalcy. Oral Surg Oral Med Oral Pathol 1984;
58(3):272–9.

39. Hoppenreijs TJ. Evaluation of condylar resorption
before and after orthognathic surgery. Semin Orthod
2013;19(2):106–15.

40. Hwang SJ, Haers PE, Zimmermann A, et al. Surgical
risk factors for condylar resorption after orthognathic
surgery. Oral Surg Oral Med Oral Pathol Oral Radiol
Endod 2000;89(5):542–52.

41. Wolford LM, Reiche-Fischel O, Mehra P. Changes
in temporomandibular joint dysfunction after orthognathic surgery. J Oral Maxillofac Surg 2003;61(6):
655–60 [discussion: 661].

42. Gomes LR, Gomes M, Jung B, et al. Diagnostic index of three-dimensional osteoarthritic
changes in temporomandibular joint condylar
morphology. J Med Imaging (Bellingham) 2015;
2(3):034501.

43. Gomes LR, Gomes MR, Gonçalves JR, et al. Cone
beam computed tomography-based models versus
multislice spiral computed tomography-based
models for assessing condylar morphology. Oral
Surg Oral Med Oral Pathol Oral Radiol 2016;
121(1):96–105.

44. Borstlap WA, Stoelinga PJ, Hoppenreijs TJ, et al.
Stabilisation of sagittal split advancement osteotomies with miniplates: a prospective, multicentre
study with two-year follow-up. Part III–condylar remodelling and resorption. Int J Oral Maxillofac
Surg 2004;33(7):649–55.

45. de Leeuw R, Boering G, Stegenga B, et al. Radiographic signs of temporomandibular joint osteoarthrosis and internal derangement 30 years after
nonsurgical treatment. Oral Surg Oral Med Oral
Pathol Oral Radiol Endod 1995;79(3):382–92.

46. Abramowicz S, Cheon JE, Kim S, et al. Magnetic
resonance imaging of the temporomandibular joints
in children with arthritis. J Oral Maxillofac Surg 2011;
69(9):2321–8.

47. Cisneros GJ, Kaban LB. Computerized skeletal scintigraphy for assessment of mandibular asymmetry.
J Oral Maxillofac Surg 1984;42(8):513–20.

48. Pogrel MA, Kopf J, Dodson TB, et al. A comparison
of single-photon emission computed tomography
and planar imaging for quantitative skeletal scintigraphy of the mandibular condyle. Oral Surg Oral
Med Oral Pathol Oral Radiol Endod 1995;80(2):
226–31.

49. Pripatnanont P, Vittayakittipong P, Markmanee U,
et al. The use of SPECT to evaluate growth cessation
of the mandible in unilateral condylar hyperplasia.
Int J Oral Maxillofac Surg 2005;34(4):364–8.

50. Teitelbaum J, Bouletreau P, Breton P, et al. Is
condylar resorption a contra-indication for surgery?
Rev Stomatol Chir Maxillofac 2007;108(3):193–200
[in French].

51. Gunson MJ, Arnett GW, Milam SB. Pathophysiology
and pharmacologic control of osseous mandibular
condylar resorption. J Oral Maxillofac Surg 2012;
70(8):1918–34.

52. Wolford LM. Clinical indications for simultaneous
TMJ and orthognathic surgery. Cranio 2007;25(4):
273–82.

53. Mehra P, Nadershah M, Chigurupati R. Is alloplastic
temporomandibular joint reconstruction a viable option in the surgical management of adult patients

with idiopathic condylar resorption? J Oral Maxillofac Surg 2016;74(10):2044–54.

54. Schendel SA, Tulasne JF, Linck DW 3rd. Idiopathic condylar resorption and micrognathia: the case for distraction osteogenesis. J Oral Maxillofac Surg 2007;65(8):1610–6.

55. Coleta KE, Wolford LM, Gonçalves JR, et al. Maxillomandibular counter-clockwise rotation and mandibular advancement with TMJ Concepts total joint prostheses: part II–airway changes and stability. Int J Oral Maxillofac Surg 2009;38(3):228–35.

56. Mehra P, Arya V, Henry C. Temporomandibular joint condylar osteochondroma: complete condylectomy and joint replacement versus low condylectomy and joint preservation. J Oral Maxillofac Surg 2016; 74(5):911–25.

57. Mercuri LG. Osteoarthritis, osteoarthrosis, and idiopathic condylar resorption. Oral Maxillofac Surg Clin North Am 2008;20(2):169–83, v–vi.

58. Nadershah M, Mehra P. Orthognathic surgery in the presence of temporomandibular dysfunction: what happens next? Oral Maxillofac Surg Clin North Am 2015;27(1):11–26.

59. Mercuri LG, Edibam NR, Giobbie-Hurder A. Fourteen-year follow-up of a patient-fitted total temporomandibular joint reconstruction system. J Oral Maxillofac Surg 2007;65(6):1140–8.

60. Wolford LM, Mercuri LG, Schneiderman ED, et al. Twenty-year follow-up study on a patient-fitted temporomandibular joint prosthesis: the Techmedica/TMJ Concepts device. J Oral Maxillofac Surg 2015;73(5):952–60.

The Role of Stress in the Etiology of Oral Parafunction and Myofascial Pain

Richard Ohrbach, DDS, PhD[a],*, Ambra Michelotti, BSc, DDS[b]

KEYWORDS

- Stress • Temporomandibular disorders • Oral parafunction • Behavior • Pain • Myofascial pain

KEY POINTS

- Oral parafunction during waking comprises many possible behaviors beyond those based on tooth contact, and awake parafunction must be distinguished from sleeping parafunction.
- Stress, parafunction, and myofascial pain are complex and comprise an assumed causal chain. However, how each component is measured can lead to different conclusions about causation.
- Experimental stress increases oral parafunction and, in turn, pain. Psychosocial stress is often accompanied by anxiety, hypervigilance, and somatosensory amplification, which also contribute to pain.
- Longitudinal research studies indicate that a high amount of awake parafunction is strongly associated with the first episode of masticatory myofascial pain.
- Successful assessment and treatment of awake oral parafunction requires consideration of multiple factors, and the causal pathway may be simple for some individuals but complex for others.

INTRODUCTION

Early publications about painful musculoskeletal disorders of the jaw, with varying levels of evidence, often referred to stress, oral parafunction, or both in combination as important contributors to these disorders.[1–3] After that early literature, a now-classic summary in 1973 proposed 4 major theories underlying the etiology of temporomandibular disorders (TMDs), two of which were psychological and psychophysiologic.[4] Subsequently, the biopsychosocial framework for considering TMDs became dominant,[5,6] with stress, oral parafunction, and TMD pain remaining an active theory. Yet, across this entire period, every element of this proposed set of causal relationships has remained challenging in terms of definition and, consequently, measurement and meaningfulness. Varying definitions and measurements have influenced the available evidence since the early texts to the present, contributing to substantial controversy. The goal of this article is to review how stress may affect behavior and TMD pain. It examines the causal hypothesis and addresses it via 3 perspectives within the existing literature: concepts, definitions, and measures; experimental studies; and observational studies. Given the complexity of the topic and the available space for this article, the literature has been selectively referenced to highlight areas of convergence as well as divergence.

Disclosure: The authors have nothing to disclose.
[a] Department of Oral Diagnostic Sciences, University at Buffalo School of Dental Medicine, 355 Squire, Buffalo, NY 14214, USA; [b] Department of Neuroscience, Reproductive Sciences and Oral Sciences, Section of Orthodontics, University of Naples Federico II, Via Pansini 5-80131-Naples, Italy
* Corresponding author.
E-mail address: ohrbach@buffalo.edu

Oral Maxillofacial Surg Clin N Am 30 (2018) 369–379
https://doi.org/10.1016/j.coms.2018.04.011
1042-3699/18/© 2018 Elsevier Inc. All rights reserved.

CONCEPTS, DEFINITIONS, AND MEASURES
Stress

Psychological stress, a process that includes both stressors as stimuli and stress reactivity as the consequence, is clearly implicated in TMDs. For example, stressful life events are highly prevalent in individuals with TMD.[7–9] Such patients report that stress initiates, exacerbates, or perpetuates their pain,[10] and stress affects treatment responsiveness.[11–13] In these examples, stress acts through multiple mechanisms that coexist with the mechanism of interest for the present article: the self-report of stress leading to a specific physiologic response pattern. The stress response system is an initially adaptive, but chronically nonadaptive, physiologic process. It is initiated by, but coextensive with, either a physiologic burden (eg, cancer pain) or psychosocial context (eg, job stress), the result of a transaction between individual coping resources and environmental demands.[14] Much controversy surrounding stress and TMD pain emerges from different conceptions of stress, its measurement, and the time base.[15–17]

The most commonly used measurement scale that incorporates the transactional aspect of the stress response is the Perceived Stress Scale (PSS), which has strong validity and usefulness.[18,19] Stress is also measured as a single question such as, "Please rate your average level of stress," using anchors of 0 (no stress) and 10 (maximal stress).[20] Single item scales are particularly useful in clinical settings and have high face validity.

Oral Parafunction

Oral, masticatory, and facial behaviors that do not serve any functional purpose are broadly termed oral parafunction.[21] These behaviors are usually harmless but, when the frequency or forces exceed some physiologic tolerance, they seem to cause harmful effects on muscles and joints[22–24] and are presumed to be important initiating and perpetuating factors in TMDs. These behaviors occur during either sleeping or waking hours. The term bruxism is inconsistently used, variously referring to any of the following: grinding of the teeth only during sleep, grinding of the teeth during sleep and when awake, grinding and clenching of the teeth only during sleep, and grinding and clenching of the teeth during sleep and when awake. Current evidence favors different mechanisms underlying sleep versus awake parafunctional behaviors, and consequently combining them helps neither understanding nor clinical management.

Parafunctional behaviors of tooth grinding or clenching that occur during sleep are currently considered a sleep disorder. Whether stress substantially affects the episodic onset of sleep bruxism is presently poorly understood, and whether sleep bruxism is even associated with pain is currently controversial.[25] Sleep bruxism is not further addressed herein, and excellent material can be found elsewhere.[26–30]

Awake parafunctional behaviors include tooth clenching, bracing, and tapping, as well as tongue pushing, among many others, and are the focus of the rest of this article. The measurement of such behaviors, however, has traditionally been very difficult, in large part because they typically occur outside the individual's awareness.[31] A simple inquiry regarding unconscious behaviors often leads to potentially false-negative reports.[32] Consequently, current evidence suggests that associations reported to date between, for example, stress and parafunction are likely underestimates.[33] In addition, research has focused primarily on grinding and clenching, and has most often ignored the wider range of oral behaviors. For example, 52% of patients with TMD pain report tooth-contacting behaviors that are distinguished from clenching.[34] Also, including other parafunctional behaviors, such as tongue bracing or tongue position, will increase the proportion of individuals reporting behaviors of potential importance.

Adequate parafunctional measurement methods include ambulatory electromyography in research contexts, but most often rely on self-observations using a paper symptom log, time-based prompting[35] such as within experience sampling methods (ESM),[36] or a checklist for rating each of multiple behaviors. The last approach is currently available as the Oral Behaviors Checklist (OBC),[21,37] and is part of the Diagnostic Criteria for Temporomandibular Disorders.[38] The OBC invites the respondent to consider whether each behavior falls into their repertoire. The OBC (score range from 0 to 84) has good test–retest reliability.[39,40] When highlighting uniqueness as well as similarity, item correlations range from r = 0.39 to 0.89.[39] Concurrent validity is r = 0.76, using an alternative oral parafunction questionnaire,[39] demonstrating acceptable operationalization of this complex construct.

Completing a self-report instrument in the clinic as a valid measure of parafunctional behaviors that are typically unconscious may seem improbable. To assess the ecologic validity of the OBC, an adapted version was administered before and after an approximately 7-day field ESM study (see Observational Studies section), in which subjects were randomly prompted up to 14 times per day and asked at each prompt to report on each of 10 different oral parafunctional behaviors. High variability regarding which behavior(s) occurred on which day was noted, yet recall of the different behaviors on the OBC at the end of the ESM period was reliable. The extent of behaviors reported via the OBC exhibit a linear relationship with the extent of behaviors recorded in the field. The predictive value of the OBC total score was measured as the area under the receiver operating curve (range, 0–1), which was 0.88 for the ESM-based study score.[40] Excellent measurement reliability[40] and semantic validity[21,37] provide evidence of a psychometrically sufficient instrument capable of measuring behaviors that typically occur unconsciously.

Myofascial Pain

Multiple diagnostic labels exist for masticatory muscle pain, perhaps because of limited evidence for peripheral pathophysiology. Myalgia is often used to denote simple local pain and myofascial pain to denote referred pain.[38] However, the term myofascial pain is also often considered inclusive of local pain. Classically, myofascial pain includes trigger points, taut bands, and pain referral as defining characteristics; local trauma and overuse behaviors as primary triggers; and overuse behaviors as a perpetuating factor.[41] However, poor evidence regarding trigger points and taut bands, poor stability of findings, and difficulty with examiner reliability surround the concept of myofascial pain.[42–46]

Myofascial pain, purported to represent a disorder of peripheral tissues,[41] may be primarily a central phenomenon.[47] However, peripheral nociceptive mediators[48] and electrical correlates of abnormal muscle activity[49,50] provide important support for local mechanisms. Myofascial pain is often simply used to refer to benign muscle pain accompanied by hyperalgesia or pain from functioning, in part because the critically defining characteristics of the chronic benign muscle pain syndromes do not differ so much across the differently labeled disorders (eg, myalgia vs myofascial pain).[6,38] Diagnostic reliability and validity are well-established for this disorder when the examination is highly structured, permitting generalization from many research studies.[38,51] Myofascial pain should be considered a disorder that may be related to muscle overuse, such as previously described under oral parafunction.

Etiology

Given the complex clinical presentation and absence of pathognomonic signs for most chronic pain disorders, the identification of etiologic factors and mechanisms is an especially critical goal. Etiology implicitly involves a clear pathway underlying causation of a disease, that expectation aligning with the classic necessary and sufficient criteria for factors related to disease onset.[52] However, for chronic disorders or complex disorders (and TMDs can be both), etiology considered as a single factor meeting the necessary and sufficient criteria is a misplaced concept, replaced instead by a mosaic of multiple risk determinants unfolding and changing across time and resulting in a raising or lowering of the threshold by which the disease of interest may occur.[53,54] The term etiology should, therefore, be considered in a very broad context, perhaps as the association between 2 variables, one occurring before the other and thereby meeting the criterion of a time sequence for a causal relationship.

EXPERIMENTAL STUDIES

The experimental research is largely oriented toward testing only 1 part of the causal chain in a given study. The following sections describe each part of the causal chain.

Stress and Oral Parafunction

The effect of stress on masticatory muscle activity—a psychophysiologic theory—was proposed by Moulton,[55] based on clinical observation but not tested until several decades later via experimental manipulation of a stress experience and measurement of masticatory muscle activity as an indicator of oral parafunction. In response to imagined stress in the laboratory, individuals with myofascial pain exhibit greater masticatory muscle activity compared with healthy controls and individuals with chronic back pain. However, the magnitude of the increase in masticatory muscle activity from before to after the stress was only about 1 microvolt.[56] Of note, in terms of a specific vulnerability with regard to how stress affects the motor system of persons with TMD, their biceps muscle did not respond to the stress imagery. These experimental results differ from those reported in another classic study where masticatory muscle activity was measured in relation to reaction time in avoiding an electrical shock. Individuals with myofascial pain exhibited less muscle activity during the trials compared with healthy controls.[17] This study has often been used to demonstrate that stress does not contribute to parafunctional behaviors as measured by masticatory muscle activity. However, the method of inducing experimental stress substantially influences the pattern of muscle activity and the self-report of stimulus-related stress,[16] indicating variation in the degree of ecologic validity of experimental studies evaluating the stress–hyperactivity relationship. Those studies with higher ecological validity, inducing the types of mental states that are most frequently reported by individuals with persistent pain, show a similar pattern of small but reliable increases in muscle activity in response to induced stress.

The stereotypical pattern of masticatory muscle response exhibited by those with a TMD is indicative of parafunctional behavior responses, although clearly an increase of about 1 μV in masticatory muscle activity, although significant, points to a minimal effect. Such small increases have been questioned with regard to how they could be causal for a pain disorder when the nervous system acts to inhibit such behavior in response to nociception.[57] As reviewed and accompanied by peer commentary,[15,58] persistent drive to the motor system via recurrent stress, accompanied by persistent albeit low-level tonic contractions of the masticatory muscles, distinguishes those with and without myofascial pain. Further evidence demonstrates the full impact of motivation: if 1 motor pattern produces pain, alternative strategies are developed to change the motor group responsible for a given movement.[59]

Oral Parafunction and Myofascial Pain

A significant association between daytime clenching and myofascial pain in the masticatory muscles has been demonstrated by self-report[22,23] and objective recordings.[60–62] For example, pain-free individuals who clenched for 20 minutes per day for 8 days in a laboratory reported significantly more pain at the end of the study than at the beginning.[63] Similarly, sustained low-level tooth clenching induced soreness in the elevator jaw muscles in healthy subjects.[64] Finally, myofascial pain symptoms decreased after treatment reducing parafunctional behavior.[65] In contrast, other studies claim that the contribution of parafunction to myofascial pain may be limited,[39,66,67] but such findings may reflect the difficulty in identifying the presence of waking-state oral parafunction in the natural environment.[21]

Objective and more reliable measurements based on electromyographic assessments[68] better assess the possible relation between daytime clenching and TMD pain. The frequency of daytime clenching episodes (defined as >10% of the maximum voluntary contraction [MVC]) is about 5-fold greater in individuals with myofascial pain compared with healthy controls.[69] More specifically, individuals with myofascial pain have fewer clenching episodes (4%) at 10% to 20% of MVC and more episodes (43%) at 30% or higher of MVC. In contrast, healthy controls have more episodes (41%) at 10% to 20% of MVC and fewer episodes (21%) at 30% or higher of MVC. Moreover,

the cumulative duration of the clenching episodes is greater in those with myofascial pain compared with healthy controls. These data suggest that individuals with myofascial pain have a high frequency of parafunctional behaviors of different intensity, such that myofascial pain might be a manifestation of muscle overload owing to an alternating pattern of high- and low-level muscle contraction episodes. Although speculative, the metabolic demand of such muscular exercise may not be satisfied when there is myofascial pain, thus, leading to muscle fatigue and increased pain. For example, delayed onset muscular soreness occurred in healthy subjects after concentric and eccentric muscle contractions of different intensity.[24] Blood flow decreased during the contractions, implying that metabolite accumulation may contribute to peripheral nociception and pain. However, further studies are needed to test the specific mechanisms of delayed onset masticatory myofascial pain.

Stress and Myofascial Pain

In addition to research focused on the stress-induced motor responses of the masticatory muscles,[57,70] a key established mechanism by which psychological stress contributes to TMD pain is the direct effect of stress and anxiety on pain sensitivity.[71–73] For example, academic examinations, a valid, naturally stressful, condition,[74,75] decreased the pressure pain thresholds of the masticatory muscles and the Achilles tendon in symptom-free dental students in relation to a significant elevation of stress and state anxiety ratings on the day of the examination.[76] Multiple parts of the central and peripheral nervous systems are activated during stress. Stress and anxiety increase sympathetic activity and the release of epinephrine at the sympathetic terminals, which may sensitize or directly activate the nociceptors.[77] The ascending reticular activating system also may play a role in the onset, maintenance, or both of chronic pain.[78] Impairment of the central nervous system pain regulatory systems, including the ascending reticular activating system, may also be responsible for the generalized enhanced pain sensitivity found in patients with TMD.[79]

According to the perceptual disruption theory,[73] stress and anxiety contribute to alterations in pain perception by disinhibiting the central nervous system structures involved in the regulation of attention (eg, ascending reticular activating system). This disruption can result in hypervigilance, which is associated with an increased attention to, or amplification of, nociceptive stimuli during a long-lasting stressful condition, and somatosensory amplification, which refers to how maladaptive cognitions can lead to heightened pain perception.[80–82] Somatosensory amplification also refers to the tendency to perceive a given somatic sensation as intense, noxious, and disturbing,[80] and somatosensory amplification is correlated with several indices of general distress, including anxious and depressive symptoms.[83–85]

In summary, stress induces motor responses of the masticatory muscles in both individuals with and without myofascial pain, but individuals with myofascial pain exhibit greater psychological and emotional distress than those without it. Also, individuals with myofascial pain exhibit a greater frequency and duration of parafunctional behavior compared with individuals without myofascial pain, and oral parafunction may contribute substantially to the myofascial pain. Furthermore, a reduction of awake oral parafunction reduces myofascial pain, further evidence of a causal relationship.

OBSERVATIONAL STUDIES

Three types of observational studies have examined the role of stress on oral parafunction and myofascial pain and help to bridge the critical gaps in the experimental studies.

Experimental Sampling Methods

ESM refers to high-density within-subject data collection.[86] By randomly sampling an individual's behavior throughout an observation period, such as multiple days or weeks, a better estimate of parafunctional behaviors across time can be obtained, which is important for those behaviors that are often unconscious. Causal processes among variables also can be better explored through time-lag modeling.

When ESM methodology was used to collect data on stress, masticatory muscle tension, tooth contact (a composite of time and intensity), and jaw pain every 2 hours via prompting by a pager over multiple days, those with chronic myofascial pain (with or without arthralgia) reported significantly greater pain, muscle tension, tooth contact, and stress. The latter 3 variables accounted for 69% of the variability (representing a reasonable model fit) in reported pain, leading to the conclusion that stress and parafunctional behaviors predict future jaw muscle pain.[87] Although individuals without TMD pain also report some level of oral parafunction, those with TMD pain report significantly higher levels. However, are the behaviors the result of the pain, the cause, or perhaps both?

The research described herein suggests that a bidirectional pathway exists between oral parafunction and chronic myofascial pain. Based on longitudinal multilevel modeling of 7023 observations from 171 individuals, distress and muscle tension contribute to myofascial pain better than pain contributes to distress, changes in distress predict tension better than tension predicts distress, and muscle tension (as a surrogate of parafunction, as described elsewhere in this article) mediates the effect of distress on myofascial pain.[33] Note that these results point to both a dominant pathway and a weaker reverse pathway. Overall, these results support a general causal chain linking stress to parafunctional behaviors to myofascial pain, although the presence of reverse pathways is consistent with the lack of simple causal relationships for complex disorders.

Do parafunctional behaviors, especially of low intensity, occur at a frequency sufficient to actually impact on either resting muscle length or the character of muscle fibers and thereby set the stage for the development of some type of myofascial pain? Early experimental studies used extremely high occlusal forces during clenching or bruxing to cause pain,[88] but such studies are not ecologically valid. In contrast, low-intensity activity of pain disorder-specific muscles occurs in response to experimental stress, indicating that reacting to stress via the body clearly differs in those with chronic pain.[70] But does this also indicate that parafunctional behavior is a valid mediating variable for the muscle pain? What kind of mechanism might account for the relationship when low-level forces potentially have insufficient energy to cause any type of muscle fiber change? Moreover, wouldn't any pain produced result in immediate inhibition of that behavior? Motivational drive can overcome inhibitory controls.[59]

In examining the actual frequency of oral parafunctional behaviors, regardless of whether stress is the proximal trigger, individuals with myofascial pain reported a median of 35% of waking time (range, 27%–41%) devoted to nonfunctional tooth contact, compared with nonpain individuals who reported a median of 9% (range, 2%–14%).[60] Nonfunctional contact was similar across days, consistent with the findings reported herein. When these findings were replicated, those with myofascial pain reported nonfunctional tooth contact during about 35% of the ESM prompts, whereas those without myofascial pain reported about 10%.[34] These findings point to how greatly frequent but low-level parafunctional behavior might contribute to the development, maintenance, or both, of myofascial pain. When stress is considered, those with TMD pain also reported significantly higher PSS scores, although these scores did not correlate with the frequency of nonfunctional tooth contact,[60] implying that multiple mechanisms may exist that lead to the particular behaviors at a given time.

Cross-Sectional Studies

Cross-sectional studies are less informative, but highly prevalent in the literature. When nursing students with TMD pain, temporomandibular joint disorders, or both, were compared with individuals without TMD, both recent life events (representing psychosocial stress) and parafunctional behaviors (using an early prototype of the OBC) were positively (but weakly) associated with each other and with painful TMD (determined via a continuous measure), but not in those without pain.[89] However, a representative example of a cross-sectional study with an opposite finding illustrates why ESM investigations are critical for this area of research. In 251 adults with TMD, their pain and the clinical variables of oral parafunction, stressors, distress, arousal, and sleep problems were recorded at the initial consultation visit. All clinical variables were associated with pain symptoms except oral parafunction, although emotional arousal was significantly associated with such symptoms.[90] The authors noted that perhaps the patients did not accurately report their level of oral parafunction. Although the oral parafunction checklist was a 12-item precursor of the items in the OBC and, therefore, had similar content validity, its response options were binary. This may have 2 consequences: reduced respondent engagement in the self-testing of the items for lack of familiarity and reduced reporting of parafunctional behavior owing to the all-or-none response scale.

Data from ESM-based studies have been replicated in simpler study designs; cross-methods approaches increase the validity of these findings. In 235 patients seeking care at a general medical clinic, those with head pain reported that clenching occurred during 41% of the day (standard deviation, 33%), and simple tooth contact occurred during 65% (standard deviation, 30%), contrasting with 17% (standard deviation, 25%) and 40% (standard deviation, 31%), respectively, in those without head pain.[63] This pattern parallels those from the ESM study previously described in which both clenching and tooth contact were significantly associated with head pain.[34]

In the large scale Orofacial Pain Prospective Evaluation and Risk Assessment (OPPERA) study,[91] individuals with chronic TMD pain, in contrast with those with no history of TMD pain, reported a high frequency of multiple oral parafunctional behaviors.[92] The authors noted that this suggested a bidirectional relationship between the behaviors and having pain or other comorbid psychological states such as stress. Stress, as measured by the PSS, also exhibited a standardized odds ratio (ie, per 1 unit of standard deviation of the predictor variable) of 1.5 for association with chronic TMD pain.[93] These findings are similar to those previously reported from a survey in which the odds ratio for an association with facial pain was 8.6 for awake clenching and 1.7 for high stress.[94]

Prospective Studies

Prospective studies of the relationship between stress, parafunction, and myofascial pain are rare. As a second part of the OPPERA study, the authors assessed the predictive power of the OBC as a measure of oral parafunction in the development of first onset TMD pain (myofascial pain, arthralgia). Oral behaviors, with a score of 25 or more, compared with a score of 16 or less, are associated with a hazard ratio of 1.75 in predicting the first onset of TMD pain. In other words, individuals with no history of TMD pain, but with an OBC score of 25 or greater, are 75% more likely to develop new TMD pain than individuals with a score of 16 or less. These results, although they highlight the early role of oral parafunction in myofascial pain onset, help little with regard to understanding potential mechanisms and rather point to future research areas.

In summary, current evidence indicates that moment-to-moment stress experience leads to a reactive behavior, such as oral parafunction in individuals with that vulnerability. Low to moderate levels of oral parafunction are benign, but high levels contribute substantially to the onset of myofascial pain. High-level parafunction is composed of both great frequency and multiple types of behavior. Pain persistence seems to act as a further stressor, leading to yet greater levels of oral parafunction.

PROPOSED MECHANISMS

The available literature suggests that stress reactivity is associated with awake oral parafunctional behaviors and that these behaviors are associated with myofascial pain. However, this same literature also suggests that the mechanisms underlying causal relations among these 3 variables may involve multiple pathways. These include oral parafunction mediating between stress and pain, oral parafunction as a trait behavior contributing to both pain and stress, oral parafunction as a consequence of pain as a stressor, and awake parafunction as a form of guarding within the fear–avoidance model.[95,96] The central importance of pain must be considered in these pathways. For example, individuals with TMD pain report greater psychological and emotional distress than those without pain, and patients with chronic TMD pain report higher levels of somatoform disorders and mood disorders (eg, depression) than patients with acute TMD pain.[93,97] In contrast, individuals with intracapsular temporomandibular joint disorders, but without pain, often report lower levels of emotional distress[98] and parafunctional behaviors have less impact on such disorders.[22,89] In addition, individuals with persistent pain are more likely to have upregulation of sympathetic drive,[99] which may also lead directly to motor cortex activation. In short, the mechanisms associated with oral parafunction point to a complex process, which should not be surprising given that behavior is the manifestation of a final pathway that is also often multiply determined, and given that TMD is a complex disorder.

The classic concept underlying the etiology of myofascial pain has included a simple direct effect of overuse behaviors that effectively reduce muscle fiber length and thereby promote the development of trigger points and taut bands as part of the process leading to myofascial pain.[41] This model was elaborated to incorporate the psychophysiologic data associated with awake oral parafunction as 1 type of overuse behavior.[15] This simple mechanical-type model is not disproved by any of the studies described in this article, but the mechanisms associated with oral parafunction can be substantially enriched, particularly in relation to the central importance of pain and anxiety. Cofactors of anxiety and somatosensory amplification seem to differentially affect pain sensitivity between the trigeminal and extratrigeminal regions, and higher levels of oral parafunctional behavior occur in response to regional nociception in the presence of these cofactors.[100] Oral parafunction may occur as a protective or guarding behavior, such as described by the fear–avoidance model, and oral parafunction may, therefore, also be associated with the critical nodes of that model: avoidance of function owing to threat, a continued decrease in pain threshold with attempted function, regional muscle atrophy, depressed mood, and pain persistence.[96] The potentially threatening stimulus is pain, and anxious individuals often exhibit both hypervigilance (increased scanning of the environment and self) as well as a pronounced attentional bias toward potential threat.[81,101,102] When the central nervous system has been upregulated with regard to

somatosensory amplification,[103] such anxiety and attentional bias is even more oriented toward a persistent focus on potential painful sensation.[104,105] State anxiety, as one aspect of psychosocial stress, may be a temporally proximal trigger for parafunctional episodes, but because anxious individuals are more vigilant and have a lasting tendency to direct their attention to threat,[106] parafunction then becomes a potential coping mechanism, albeit one that may help with regulating emotion rather than altering the stressful situation.

Consequently, the combination of hypervigilance and anxiety seems to be additive, nonadaptive, and persistent beyond the stress episodes. Although these assumptions probably point to causal relationships between anxiety, somatosensory amplification, and increased pain perception, heightened body awareness (ie, increased somatosensory amplification and hypervigilance) and anxiety also could be a consequence of heightened sensitivity to pain stimuli. Individual differences in this process could also be due to genetic influences.[107] Individuals with myofascial pain have high levels of somatosensory amplification[108] that are characterized by a bodily hypervigilance to unpleasant sensations,[80] and in individuals with high parafunction, different levels of somatosensory amplification might account for the differing extent of subjective complaints. In contrast, individuals with a low amount of parafunction who have low trait anxiety may have an avoidant attention style that allows them to shift their attention away from potential threat and thereby not develop any significant level of myofascial pain.

SUMMARY

The available evidence supports a causal chain of stress, awake oral parafunction, and myofascial pain. However, this sequence seems to coexist with other mechanisms that link stress and other psychological processes directly with myofascial pain. Affective distress can directly contribute to myofascial pain, and individuals with hypervigilance in conjunction with high levels of stress reactivity as well as anxiety are more vulnerable to threat from regional pain and to the use of parafunction as a coping method for that threat. Anxiety, stress, somatosensory amplification, and increased pain perception may represent a critical set of risk determinants that increase the probability for developing myofascial pain. Awake oral parafunction is an established risk determinant for myofascial pain onset and persistence. It may contribute in both a direct manner with regard to altering muscle fiber length and thereby set the stage for an experience of bodily threat owing to altered function, as well as in an indirect manner as a potentially nonadaptive coping method.

REFERENCES

1. Schwartz LL. Pain associated with the temporomandibular joint. J Am Dent Assoc 1955;4:393–7.
2. Shore NA. Occlusal equilibration and temporomandibular joint dysfunction. Philadelphia: Lippincott; 1959.
3. Laskin DM. Etiology of the pain-dysfunction syndrome. J Am Dent Assoc 1969;79:147–53.
4. De Boever JA. Functional disturbances of temporomandibular joints. Oral Sci Rev 1973;2: 100–17.
5. Dworkin SF. Illness behavior and dysfunction: review of concepts and application to chronic pain. Can J Physiol Pharmacol 1991;69:662–71.
6. Dworkin SF, LeResche L. Research diagnostic criteria for temporomandibular disorders: review, criteria, examinations and specifications, critique. J Craniomandib Disord 1992;6(4):301–55.
7. Rugh J, Solberg W. Psychological implications in temporomandibular pain and dysfunction. Oral Sci Rev 1976;7:3–30.
8. Speculand B, Hughes AO, Goss AN. Role of recent stressful life events experience in the onset of TMJ dysfunction pain. Community Dent Oral Epidemiol 1984;12:197–202.
9. Dahlström L. Psychometrics in temporomandibular disorders: an overview. Acta Odontol Scand 1993; 51(6):339–52.
10. Suvinen TI, Hanes KR, Gerschman JA, et al. Psychophysical subtypes of temporomandibular disorders. J Orofac Pain 1997;11(3):200–5.
11. Widerstrom-Noga E, Dyrehag LE, Borglum-Jensen L, et al. Pain threshold responses to two different modes of sensory stimulation in patients with orofacial muscular pain: psychologic considerations. J Orofac Pain 1998;12(1):27–34.
12. Fricton JR, Olsen T. Predictors of outcome for treatment of temporomandibular disorders. J Orofac Pain 1996;10(1):54–65.
13. de Leeuw JR, Ros WJ, Steenks MH, et al. Craniomandibular dysfunction: patient characteristics related to treatment outcome. J Oral Rehabil 1994;21(6):667–78.
14. Lazarus RS, Folkman S. Stress, appraisal, and coping. New York: Springer Publishing Company; 1984.
15. Ohrbach R, McCall WD Jr. The stress-hyperactivity-pain theory of myogenic pain: proposal for a revised theory. Pain Forum 1996;5:51–66.
16. Ohrbach R, Blascovich J, Gale EN, et al. Psychophysiological assessment of stress in chronic pain: a comparison of stressful stimuli and response systems. J Dent Res 1998;77:1840–50.
17. Intrieri RC, Jones GE, Alcorn JD. Masseter muscle hyperactivity and myofascial pain dysfunction syndrome: a relationship under stress. J Behav Med 1994;17:479–500.
18. Cohen S, Kamarck T, Mermelstein R. A global measure of perceived stress. J Health Hum Behav 1983;24:385–96.
19. Cohen S, Williamson GM. Perceived stress in a probability sample in the United States. In: Spacapan S, Oakamp S, editors. The social psychology of health. Newburg Park (CA): Sage; 1988. p. 31–67.
20. Slade G, Sanders A, Ohrbach R, et al. COMT diplotype amplifies effect of stress on risk of temporomandibular pain. J Dent Res 2015;94(9):1187–95.
21. Ohrbach R, Markiewicz MR, McCall WD Jr. Waking-state oral parafunctional behaviors: specificity and validity as assessed by electromyography. Eur J Oral Sci 2008;116(5):438–44.
22. Michelotti A, Cioffi I, Festa P, et al. Oral parafunctions as risk factors for diagnostic TMD subgroups. J Oral Rehabil 2010;37(3):157–62.
23. Huang GJ, LeResche L, Critchlow CW, et al. Risk factors for diagnostic subgroups of painful temporomandibular disorders (TMD). J Dent Res 2002; 81(4):284–8.
24. Koutris M, Lobbezoo F, Sümer NC, et al. Is myofascial pain in temporomandibular disorder patients a manifestation of delayed-onset muscle soreness? Clin J Pain 2013;29(8):712–6.
25. Raphael KG, Sirois DA, Janal MN, et al. Sleep bruxism and myofascial temporomandibular disorders: a laboratory polysomnographic investigation. J Am Dent Assoc 2012;143(11):1223–31.
26. Manfredini D, Lobbezoo F. Relationship between bruxism and temporomandibular disorders: a systematic review of literature from 1998 to 2008. Oral Surg Oral Med Oral Pathol Oral Radiol Endod 2010;109:e26–50.
27. Manfredini D, Winocur E, Guarda-Nardini L, et al. Self-reported bruxism and temporomandibular disorders: findings from two specialized centers. J Oral Rehabil 2012;39:319–25.
28. Raphael KGJ, Sirois MN, Dubrovsky DA, et al. Validity of self-reported sleep bruxism among myofascial temporomandibular disorder patients and controls. J Oral Rehabil 2015;42(10):751–8.
29. Dumais IE, Lavigne GJ, Carra MC, et al. Could transient hypoxia be associated with rhythmic masticatory muscle activity in sleep bruxism in the absence of sleep-disordered breathing? A preliminary report. J Oral Rehabil 2015;42(11):810–8.
30. Bertazzo-Silveira E, Kruger CM, Porto De Toledo I, et al. Association between sleep bruxism and alcohol, caffeine, tobacco, and drug abuse: a

systematic review. J Am Dent Assoc 2016;147(11): 859–66.e4.

31. Glaros AG. Awareness of physiological responding under stress and nonstress conditions in temporomandibular disorders. Biofeedback Self Regul 1996;21(3):261–72.

32. Richman WL, Kiesler S, Weisband S, et al. A meta-analytic study of social desirability distortion in computer-administered questionnaires, traditional questionnaires, and interviews. J Appl Psychol 1999;84(5):754–75.

33. Glaros AG, Marszalek JM, Williams KB. Longitudinal multilevel modeling of facial pain, muscle tension, and stress. J Dent Res 2016;95(4):416–22.

34. Funato M, Ono Y, Baba K, et al. Evaluation of the non-functional tooth contact in patients with temporomandibular disorders by using newly developed electronic system. J Oral Rehabil 2014;41(3):170–6.

35. Glaros AG, Williams K, Lausten L. Diurnal variation in pain reports in temporomandibular disorder patients and control subjects. J Orofac Pain 2008; 22(2):115–21.

36. Conner TS, Tennen H, Fleeson W, et al. Experience sampling methods: a modern idiographic approach to personality research. Soc Personal Psychol Compass 2009;3(3):292–313.

37. Markiewicz MR, Ohrbach R, McCall WD Jr. Oral Behaviors Checklist: reliability of performance in targeted waking-state behaviors. J Orofac Pain 2006;20(4):306–16.

38. Schiffman E, Ohrbach R, Truelove E, et al. Diagnostic criteria for temporomandibular disorders (DC/TMD) for clinical and research applications: recommendations of the international RDC/TMD consortium network and orofacial pain special interest group. J Oral Facial Pain Headache 2014; 28(1):6–27.

39. van der Muelen MJ, Lobbezoo F, Aartman IH, et al. Validity of the oral behaviours checklist: correlations between OBC scores and intensity of facial pain. J Oral Rehabil 2014;41(2):115–21.

40. Kaplan SEF, Ohrbach R. Self-report of waking-state oral parafunctional behaviors in the natural environment. J Oral Facial Pain Headache 2016;30:107–19.

41. Travell JG, Simons DG. Myofascial pain and dysfunction: the trigger point manual. Baltimore (MD): Williams and Wilkins; 1983.

42. Dommerholt J, Gerwin RD. A critical evaluation of Quintner et al: missing the point. J Bodyw Mov Ther 2015;19(2):193–204.

43. Quintner JL, Bove GM, Cohen ML. A critical evaluation of the trigger point phenomenon. Rheumatology 2014;54(3):392–9.

44. Cohen M, Quintner J. The clinical conversation about pain: tensions between the lived experience and the biomedical model. In: Fernandez J, editor. Making Sense of Pain: Critical and Interdisciplinary Perspectives. Oxford, England: Inter-Disciplinary Press; 2010. p. 85–100.

45. Cohen M, Quintner J. The horse is dead: let myofascial pain syndrome rest in peace. Pain Med 2008;9(4):464–5.

46. Gerwin RD, Shannon S, Hong C-Z, et al. Interrater reliability in myofascial trigger point examination. Pain 1997;69:65–73.

47. Melzack R. Phantom limbs, the self and the brain. Can Psychol 1989;30:1–16.

48. Shah JP, Phillips TM, Danoff JV, et al. An in vivo microanalytical technique for measuring the local biochemical milieu of human skeletal muscle. J Appl Physiol (1985) 2005;99:1977–84.

49. Chung JW, Ohrbach R, McCall WD Jr. Effect of increased sympathetic activity on electrical activity from myofascial painful areas. Am J Phys Med Rehabil 2004;83(11):842–50.

50. Chung JW, Ohrbach R, McCall WD Jr. Characteristics of electrical activity from myofascial trigger points. Clin Neurophysiol 2006;117:2459–66.

51. John MT, Dworkin SF, Mancl LA. Reliability of clinical temporomandibular disorder diagnoses. Pain 2005;118:61–9.

52. Hill AB. The environment and disease: association or causation? Proc R Soc Med 1965;58:295–300.

53. Rothman KJ, Greenland S. Causation and causal inference in epidemiology. Am J Public Health 2005;95(S1):S144–50.

54. Galea S, Riddle M, Kaplan GA. Causal thinking and complex system approaches in epidemiology. Int J Epidemiol 2009;39(1):97–106.

55. Moulton RE. Emotional factors in non-organic temporomandibular joint pain. Dent Clin North Am 1966;609–20.

56. Flor H, Birbaumer N, Schulte W, et al. Stress-related electromyographic responses in patients with chronic temporomandibular pain. Pain 1991; 46:145–52.

57. Lund JP, Donga R, Widmer CG, et al. The pain-adaptation model: a discussion of the relationship between chronic musculoskeletal pain and motor activity. Can J Physiol Pharmacol 1991; 69:683–94.

58. Ohrbach R, McCall WD Jr. The lion at the gate. Pain Forum 1996;5:77–80.

59. Minami I, Akhter R, Albersen I, et al. Masseter motor unit recruitment is altered in experimental jaw muscle pain. J Dent Res 2013;92(2):143–8.

60. Chen C-Y, Palla S, Emi S, et al. Nonfunctional tooth contact in healthy controls and patients with myogenous facial pain. J Orofac Pain 2007;21(3): 185–93.

61. Cioffi I, Farella M, Festa P, et al. Short-term sensorimotor effects of experimental occlusal interferences on the wake-time masseter muscle activity

of females with masticatory muscle pain. J Oral Facial Pain Headache 2015;29(4):331–9.

62. Michelotti A, Cioffi I, Landino D, et al. Effects of experimental occlusal interferences in individuals reporting different levels of wake-time parafunctions. J Orofac Pain 2012;26(3):168–75.

63. Glaros AG, Williams K. Tooth contact versus clenching: oral parafunctions and facial pain. J Orofac Pain 2012;26(3):176–80.

64. Farella M, Soneda K, Vilmann A, et al. Jaw muscle soreness after tooth-clenching depends on force level. J Dent Res 2010;89(7):717–21.

65. Glaros AG, Kim-Weroha N, Lausten L, et al. Comparison of habit reversal and a behaviorally-modified dental treatment for temporomandibular disorders: a pilot investigation. Appl Psychophysiol Biofeedback 2007;32(3):149–54.

66. Velly AM, Gornitsky M, Philippe P. Contributing factors to chronic myofascial pain: a case-control study. Pain 2003;103:491–500.

67. van der Meulen MJ, Lobbezoo F, Aartman IHA, et al. Self-reported oral parafunctions and pain intensity in temporomandibular disorder patients. J Orofac Pain 2006;20:31–5.

68. Castroflorio T, Bracco P, Farina D. Surface electromyography in the assessment of jaw elevator muscles. J Oral Rehabil 2008;35(8):638–45.

69. Cioffi I, Landino D, Donnarumma V, et al. Frequency of daytime tooth clenching episodes in individuals affected by masticatory muscle pain and pain-free controls during standardized ability tasks. Clin Oral Investig 2016;21(4):1139–48.

70. Flor H, Turk DC. Psychophysiology of chronic pain: do chronic pain patients exhibit symptom-specific psychophysiological responses? Psychol Bull 1989;105:215–59.

71. Malow RM. The effects of induced anxiety on pain perception: a signal detection analysis. Pain 1981;11(3):397–405.

72. Rhudy JL, Meagher MW. Fear and anxiety: divergent effects on human pain thresholds. Pain 2000;84(1):65–75.

73. Cornwall A, Donderi DC. The effect of experimentally induced anxiety on the experience of pressure pain. Pain 1988;35:105–14.

74. Malarkey WB, Pearl DK, Demers LM, et al. Influence of academic stress and season on 24-hour mean concentrations of ACTH, cortisol, and β-endorphin. Psychoneuroendocrinology 1995;20(5):499–508.

75. Malarkey WB, Hall JC, Pearl DK, et al. The influence of academic stress and season on 24-hour concentrations of growth hormone and prolactin. J Clin Endocrinol Metab 1991;73(5):1089–92.

76. Michelotti A, Farella M, Tedesco A, et al. Changes in pressure-pain thresholds of the jaw muscles during a natural stressful condition in a group of symptom-free subjects. J Orofac Pain 2000;14(4):279–85.

77. Dubner R, Hargreaves KM. The neurobiology of pain and its modulation. Clin J Pain 1989;5(Suppl 2):S1–6.

78. Maixner W, Fillingim R, Booker D, et al. Sensitivity of patients with painful temporomandibular disorders to experimentally evoked pain. Pain 1995;63:341–51.

79. Reid KI, Gracely RH, Dubner RA. The influence of time, facial side, and location on pain-pressure thresholds in chronic myogenous temporomandibular disorder. J Orofac Pain 1994;8:258–65.

80. Barsky AJ. The amplification of somatic symptoms. Psychosom Med 1988;50:510–9.

81. Barsky AJ. Amplification, somatization, and somatoform disorders. Psychosomatics 1992;33:28–34.

82. Feuerstein M, Beattie P. Biobehavioral factors affecting pain and disability in low back pain: mechanisms and assessment. Phys Ther 1995;75(4):267–80.

83. Aronson KR, Barrett LF, Quigley KS. Feeling your body or feeling badly: evidence for the limited validity of the somatosensory amplification scale as an index of somatic sensitivity. J Psychosom Res 2001;51:387–94.

84. Duddu V, Isaac MK, Chaturvedi SK. Somatization, somatosensory amplification, attribution styles and illness behaviour: a review. Int Rev Psychiatry 2006;18:25–33.

85. Mantar A, Yemez B, Alkin T. The validity and reliability of the Turkish version of the anxiety sensitivity index-3. Turk Psikiyatri Derg 2010;21:225–34.

86. Stone AA, Broderick JE, Shiffman SS, et al. Understanding recall of weekly pain from a momentary assessment perspective: absolute agreement, between- and within-person consistency, and judged change in weekly pain. Pain 2004;107:61–9.

87. Glaros AG, Williams K, Lausten L. The role of parafunctions, emotions and stress in predicting facial pain. J Am Dent Assoc 2005;136:451–8.

88. Christenson LV. Effects of an occlusal splint on integrated electromyography of masseter muscle in experimental tooth clenching in man. J Oral Rehabil 1980;7:281–8.

89. Schiffman EL, Fricton JR, Haley D. The relationship of occlusion, parafunctional habits and recent life events to mandibular dysfunction in a non-patient population. J Oral Rehabil 1992;19:201–23.

90. Davis CE, Carlson CR, Studts JL, et al. Use of a structural equation model for prediction of pain symptoms in patients with orofacial pain and temporomandibular disorders. J Orofac Pain 2010;24(1):89–100.

91. Maixner W, Diatchenko L, Dubner R, et al. Orofacial pain prospective evaluation and risk assessment

study – the OPPERA study. J Pain 2011;12(11, Supplement 3):T4–11.

92. Ohrbach R, Bair E, Fillingim RB, et al. Clinical oro-facial characteristics associated with risk of first-onset TMD: the OPPERA prospective cohort study. J Pain 2013;14(12, supplement 2):T33–50.

93. Fillingim RB, Ohrbach R, Greenspan JD, et al. Potential psychosocial risk factors for chronic TMD: descriptive data and empirically identified domains from the OPPERA case-control study. J Pain 2011; 12(11, supplement 3):T46–60.

94. Goulet J-P, Lund JP, Lavigne G. Relation entre les habitudes parafonctionnelles, le stress et les symptômes associés aux désordres temporomandibulaires. In: Simard-Savoie S, editor. Actes du 9e Congrès de l'AIFRO. Montreal (Canada): Méridien; 1993. p. 139–44.

95. Glaros AG. Temporomandibular disorders and facial pain: a psychophysiological perspective. Appl Psychophysiol Biofeedback 2008;33(3): 161–71.

96. Leeuw M, Goossens ME, Linton SJ, et al. The fear-avoidance model of musculoskeletal pain: current state of scientific evidence. J Behav Med 2007; 30(1):77–94.

97. Fillingim RB, Ohrbach R, Greenspan JD, et al. Psychosocial factors associated with development of TMD: the OPPERA prospective cohort study. J Pain 2013;14(12, supplement 2):T75–90.

98. Manfredini D, di Poggio AB, Romagnoli M, et al. Mood spectrum in patients with different painful temporomandibular disorders. Cranio 2004;22(3): 234–40.

99. Sarlani E, Grace EG, Reynolds MA, et al. Sex differences in temporal summation of pain and aftersensations following repetitive noxious mechanical stimulation. Pain 2004;109:115–23.

100. Cioffi I, Michelotti A, Perrotta S, et al. Effect of somatosensory amplification and trait anxiety on experimentally induced orthodontic pain. Eur J Oral Sci 2016;124(2):127–34.

101. Benedetti F, Lanotte M, Lopiano L, et al. When words are painful: unraveling the mechanisms of the nocebo effect. Neuroscience 2007;147(2): 260–71.

102. Mathews A, May J, Mogg K, et al. Attentional bias in anxiety: selective search of defective filtering. J Abnorm Psychol 1990;99:166–73.

103. Diatchenko L, Nackley AG, Slade GD, et al. Idiopathic pain disorders - pathways of vulnerability. Pain 2006;123:226–30.

104. Ouimet AJ, Gawronski B, Dozois DJ. Cognitive vulnerability to anxiety: a review and an integrative model. Clin Psychol Rev 2009;29(6):459–70.

105. Mogg K, Bradley BP. A cognitive-motivational analysis of anxiety. Behav Res Ther 1998;36(9):809–48.

106. Eysenck MW, Derakshan N, Santos R, et al. Anxiety and cognitive performance: attentional control theory. Emotion 2007;7(2):336–53.

107. Belfer I, Segall SK, Lariviere WR, et al. Pain modality- and sex-specific effects of COMT genetic functional variants. Pain 2013;154(8):1368–76.

108. Raphael KG, Marbach JJ, Gallagher RM. Somatosensory amplification and affective inhibition are elevated in myofascial face pain. Pain Med 2000; 1(3):247–53.

Moving?

Make sure your subscription moves with you!

To notify us of your new address, find your **Clinics Account Number** (located on your mailing label above your name), and contact customer service at:

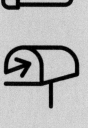

Email: journalscustomerservice-usa@elsevier.com

800-654-2452 (subscribers in the U.S. & Canada)
314-447-8871 (subscribers outside of the U.S. & Canada)

Fax number: 314-447-8029

Elsevier Health Sciences Division
Subscription Customer Service
3251 Riverport Lane
Maryland Heights, MO 63043

Printed and bound by CPI Group (UK) Ltd, Croydon, CR0 4YY

08/05/2025

01864727-0004